MS

MS

Living with Hope & Strength

VICKI CHANDLER

To order additional copies of this book, contact:
Xlibris Corporation
1-888-795-4274
www.Xlibris.com
Orders@Xlibris.com
33186

DEDICATION

This book is dedicated to all those who have prayed for me, helped me, encouraged me, ministered to me, and put up with me. First of all, I'm grateful to my husband Howie who does so much for me. Because of my disease, he has become quite a self-sufficient man in the kitchen. In addition to tenderly caring for my health needs, he shows support in countless other ways (such as faithfully praying for me just to get out of bed each morning, listening to me as I process what's going on with my body, attending MS workshops with me, going on errands, etc.). His most recent labor of love was editing the manuscript for this book.

I'm blessed to have the caring support of my sons, Chris and Rob. They are always willing to help me in any way without hesitation. I have tremendous gratitude that they have become such caring and compassionate men. I appreciate the wise counsel that they and Rob's wife, Kristie, have given me periodically.

My mother's support is a source of comfort. Her faithful prayers have helped me through many difficult times with my disease. Words cannot express the gratitude I have for all the things she does that only a mother would do (and know to do).

Several caring doctors have a part in the achievement of writing this book. I'm thankful to Dr. Nelson for urging me to write this book. His sincere love and concern for his patients led him to prompt me to take on this project. In addition, I'm grateful for Dr. Kipp and Dr. Mazlin. They are very knowledgeable, compassionate, and accessible. I'm able to do as much as I can partly due to their good care for me.

In addition, I'd like to acknowledge Donna Minnich who painted the illustration for the cover of this book. Her artistic talent and godly character captured the essence of the message I wanted to convey: Jesus is our Good Shepherd who cares for us. I'm thankful for friends like her who help me keep my focus on the Lord and not on my struggles in life.

Finally, the staff at Calvary Christian Academy shares in the victory Christ has had in my life. Their constant prayer support and concern help carry me when I'm weak. Sam and Todd show tremendous compassion. Janice is a perfect example of the type of administrator everyone with MS would want to have. She makes accommodations for me so that I'm able to continue teaching.

CONTENTS

INTRODUCTION

If you are human, you have emotions. So it's normal to have an opinion about having Multiple Sclerosis (MS) and it's normal to react emotionally. Finding out you have MS means finding out you're not in control of your life (as if anyone ever is). For me—someone who is accustomed to being in control—that was way out of my comfort zone. But my first emotion was relief. I had always been extremely tired for a long time. But 'tired' is a word everyone uses. Everybody is tired in our over scheduled society. However, people with MS experience a different level of weakness and fatigue. There's really no word to describe it. My best way I described it to my husband was, "It's TORTURE to get out of bed in the morning." I even said to him on many occasions, "Some day I'll find out I have some kind of rare disease that makes me so tired. This isn't normal tired." Well, thankfully, I did find out what disease I have. But it's not rare.

As I share my thoughts and feelings, I realize that your response might not be exactly the same as mine. Your physical journey may differ from mine. That's the nature of the disease. Your emotional response will be unlike mine, too. However, most people with MS want to have hope and don't like feeling so out of control. Everyone's spiritual journey can be the same because, "Jesus Christ is the same yesterday, today, and forever" (Hebrews 13:8). He is faithful. His Word is true. Before I share the details of my story, it's important to understand the tone of this book. It will contain descriptions of my version of the horrors of MS. Since you don't know me, you may not understand my intentions. So let me be clear. My purpose in sharing the horrible details of my story is not to complain. Nor is it to brag (in some sick way) that my situation is worse than anyone else's. The reason I will be sharing some unpleasant thoughts and details is so that you understand that I, too, truly struggle with this disease. Then, when I share God's words of hope, you cannot think, "Well, that's easy for you to say." Let me acknowledge that some of you who read this book have a more difficult journey than mine. I pray that the words of truth and hope will comfort your heart if your MS has resulted in loss of mobility, speech, vision, or bladder control.

At times in this book I'll also share humor. You might not find anything funny about MS and, therefore, might be offended. Again, it is my prayer that this book will present an uplifting perspective of how to live with MS. Certainly I realize that MS impacts tremendously on relationships, finances, and independence. But I know that the Bible says a merry heart does good like medicine (Proverbs 15:13).

In addition to sharing my awful details and humor, I'll also share anecdotes of times I cried. Normal people cry. It's actually a healthy thing to do in a sad situation as long as it doesn't lead to a pity party. There are many symptoms that all MS patients share. Fatigue is one common denominator. Usually depression is another symptom that we all experience at one time or another. Depression is so prevalent because it not only can be a symptom caused by the disease (lesions on the brain affecting emotions), it can also be a response to having the disease (a result of the disease) and a side effect of some medication (e. g., interferons and steroids). It is important to talk to your neurologist or physician about depression if you're experiencing it. There are medications that can effectively treat it. But it is equally important to talk to God in prayer about your depression. God is able to heal. He is able to provide peace and restore joy. He can create a calm countenance in the midst of a storm. Jesus calmed the waters in a storm, in Matthew 8 we read, "Now when He got into a boat, His disciples followed Him. And suddenly a great tempest arose on the sea, so that the boat was covered with the waves. But He was asleep. Then His disciples came to Him and awoke Him, saying, 'Lord, save us! We are perishing!' But He said to them, 'Why are you fearful, O you of little faith?' Then He arose and rebuked the winds and the sea. And there was a great calm. And the men marveled, saying, 'Who can this be, that even the winds and the sea obey Him?'" (Matthew 8:23-27) Yes, there will be tears, but Jesus can be the calm in the midst of your MS storm. "For with God nothing will be impossible." (Luke 1:37)

"Because He lives I can face tomorrow,
Because He lives all fear is gone,
Because I know He holds the future,
And life is worth the living, just because He lives."

CHAPTER 1

A PRESCRIPTION FOR HOPE AND STRENGTH

The Bible tells us that we will experience tribulation (a time of great affliction). Jesus said, "'These things I have spoken to you, that in Me you may have peace, in the world you will have tribulation; but be of good cheer, I have overcome the world.'" (John 16:33). As Christians, we are not without hope. We serve a living God who has given us a guidebook for life—the Bible. It contains a formula for handling stress and trials. It includes words of comfort and hope for any situation.

The following is a list of biblical strategies that offer relief from the devastation of MS. These are truths I know to be true, but often forget to follow them as I allow my focus to be on my pain or discomfort. But there are times when I am discouraged and remember to follow some of those suggestions. It's then that I find heavenly comfort. Keep this prescription from the Master Physician handy.

1) *Hope in Him, not in statistics.* People who learned of my diagnosis often shared stories of friends or relatives they knew who had MS and who were "doing fine." Even statistics are in our favor. In the National Multiple Sclerosis Society's booklet *Plaintalk—A booklet about MS for Families* it states, "We believe that two out of three people with MS remain ambulatory over their lifetimes, but many of them need a cane or other assistive device for walking, and some of them will choose a scooter or wheelchair to conserve energy." But hoping in statistics or in good self care is false hope. People get MS no matter how well they take care of themselves. As far as we know, it seems that MS afflicts people no matter what they do. In the MS Society's pamphlet *What is Multiple Sclerosis?* we read, "We do know, however, that the person who develops MS has done nothing to cause the disease or its symptoms, and could not have prevented it from occurring."

There is little comfort in knowing that someone is "doing well" with MS because of the type of alternative therapy they are using. What many people don't realize is that lesions can be forming on the brain even when the person is symptom free. That was the case with me. When I saw my MRI, I saw numerous white spots (each representing scar tissue or a lesion caused by demyelination of the nerves). When I asked if all that demyelination occurred at once or over time, my neurologist told me that it happened over a long time. So, I had MS and didn't even know it. I was always tired, but was apparently "doing fine." In their disease management consensus statement (of October 1998 and revised in October of 2002), the MS Society made a profound statement. "Serial MRI studies of individuals who are clinically in remission have demonstrated ongoing brain lesion development and atrophy despite a seemingly benign clinical course. These findings strengthen the argument for early intervention with a disease modifying agent."

Someone who is "doing fine" has a false sense of security unless their hope is in the Lord. A close friend of mine who has MS described the disease as having a time bomb in your brain. She was essentially correct. At any time those lesions that are forming could damage a nerve that would cause serious or debilitating symptoms. That's why I choose to focus on God rather than the disease. He is able to protect. I cannot stop my immune system from attacking good cells in my central nervous system, but God can. To me, my MRI was a picture of God's protection. Although lesions were forming in my brain, God protected me from having a serious exacerbation for a long time.

During the time I had MS and didn't know it, I was under considerable stress several times. While I was teaching full time, I was working toward my master's degree. At that time my father was being treated for cancer and we moved several times. But I didn't experience symptoms of an MS relapse. Another time in recent years (before my diagnosis) my oldest son, Chris, suddenly had a psychotic episode and was diagnosed with schizoaffective disorder (mental illness similar to schizophrenia). Still I didn't have an MS attack. When I helped one other administrator start a Christian school (that began with 380 students the first year and grew to over 500 in the second year), I didn't even know that I had MS. I seemed fine. In the MS Society's booklet *Living With MS* it is pointed out that, "There's no solid scientific evidence that stress either causes MS or makes it worse." It is God who protected me from having an MS relapse during those times. My hope is in Him.

2) ***Remember that God is your source of hope and strength.*** We can gain some hope and strength from good self care and treatment. But discouragement and fatigue can still plague us. We can gain much more from God. Our all powerful, all loving God offers us so much more. The Bible has a lot say about hope in the midst of affliction. It is filled with assurances.

- We can ABOUND in hope by His power. "Now may the God of hope fill you with all joy and peace in believing, that you may abound in hope by the power of the Holy Spirit." (Romans. 15:13) When your disease makes you feel out of control and hopeless, it's a wonderful reminder that we can abound in hope. We have access to unlimited hope because of His unlimited power and love.

- We do not have to lose heart. God is working His perfect plan. "Therefore we do not lose heart. Even though our outward man is perishing, yet the inward man is being renewed day by day. For our light affliction, which is but for a moment, is working for us a far more exceeding and eternal weight of glory . . ." (II Corinthians 4:16-17)

- We have a source of supernatural strength to draw upon. ". . . 'My grace is sufficient for you, for My strength is made perfect in weakness.' Therefore most gladly I will rather boast in my infirmities, that the power of Christ may rest upon me. Therefore I take pleasure in infirmities . . . for Christ's sake. For when I am weak, then I am strong." (II Corinthians 12:9-10)

- We need not lose heart or be discouraged. "I would have lost heart, unless I had believed that I would see the goodness of the Lord in the land of the living." (Psalm 27:13)

- We already have the victory because of God's love for us. "Who shall separate us from the love of Christ? Shall tribulation, or distress, or persecution, or famine, or nakedness, or peril, or sword? Yet in all these things we are more than conquerors through Him who loved us." (Romans 8:35, 37)

- We can have courage. We need not fear. "Wait on the Lord; be of good courage, and He shall strengthen your heart; wait, I say, on the Lord!" (Psalm 27:14)

- He can delight our souls in spite of the devastating disease, "In the multitude of my anxieties within me, Your comforts delight my soul." (Psalm 94:19)

- We find joy and comfort in His Word. "Your word was to me the joy and rejoicing of my heart . . ." (Jeremiah 15:16) "This is my comfort in my affliction, for Your word has given me life." (Psalm 119:50)

- He can calm us by His grace. "But may the God of all grace, who called us to His eternal glory by Christ Jesus, after you have suffered a while, perfect, establish, strengthen, and settle you." (I Peter 5:10)

3) *Remember that He is in control.* Regardless of the path the disease takes, He is in control. He is a sovereign God who has a perfect plan. His ways are not like our ways. We often don't understand why things happen to us. But we can trust that our heavenly Father has a reason for this illness. Often He uses trials to lead us to a deeper knowledge of Him. It is an opportunity to see Him work. In this book you'll find many examples of how His love was revealed to me through people. I had a chance to see His amazing power in ways I wouldn't have if I wasn't afflicted with MS. Having an MS relapse afforded me the time to read the Bible and pray. Had I not had the attack I wouldn't have had those precious times of fellowship with Him.

Sadly, in the business of life, I don't usually make the time to read the Bible. But I had time to focus on Him and know that He is in control even when things seem out of control. Often I would come across verses that reminded me that He is able to work mightily in my situation. "Behold, I am the Lord, the God of all flesh, is there anything too hard for Me?" (Jeremiah 32:27)

4) *Remember that He is faithful.* In the context of uncertainty, it's good to know that there is One who is faithful. He promises to provide all that we need. Often we need wisdom. We need to know what direction to turn in selecting a neurologist. We need to learn how much to push our bodies. We might have to decide on a job change or whether to get pregnant. God has promised that He will grant wisdom to all who ask. "If any of you lacks wisdom, let him ask of God, who gives to all liberally and without reproach, and it will be given to him." (James 1:5) He promises to provide for all our physical needs. "Look at the birds of the air, for they neither sow nor reap nor gather into barns; yet your heavenly Father feeds them. Are you not of more value than they? Therefore do not worry, saying, 'What shall we eat?' or 'What shall we drink?' or 'What shall we wear?' For after all these things the Gentiles seek. For your heavenly Father knows that you need all these things. But seek first the kingdom of God and His righteousness, and all these things shall be added to you. Therefore do not worry about tomorrow, for tomorrow will worry about its own things. Sufficient for the day is its own trouble." (Matthew 6:26, 31-34)

5) *Focus on Him primarily.* It's so easy to focus only on the disease. It can often take over lives. It's difficult or impossible to ignore. When I wake up in the morning the pain in my legs reminds me, "Oh, yea, I have MS." But then I remind myself, "Oh, yea, God is greater still." We must be resolved to renew our thinking. It is a deliberate act of faith. David, in the Old Testament, was persecuted. When he looked at his situation things looked bleak. But he chose to shift his focus to God saying often, "But God . . ."

- "Lord, how they have increased who trouble me! Many are they who rise up against me. Many are they who say of me, 'There is no help for him in God.' Selah **But** You, O Lord, are a shield for me, My glory and the One who lifts up my head." (Psalm 3:1-3)
- "They confronted me in the day of my calamity, **But** the Lord was my support." (Psalm 18:18)
- "Many are the afflictions of the righteous, **But** the Lord delivers him out of them all." (Psalm 34:19)
- "My flesh and my heart fail; **But** God is the strength of my heart and my portion forever." (Psalm 73:26)
- "I cried out to God with my voice—To God with my voice; and He gave ear to me. In the day of my trouble I sought the Lord; my hand was stretched out in the night without ceasing; my soul refused to be comforted. I remembered God, and was troubled; I complained, and my spirit was overwhelmed. Selah. You hold my eyelids open; I am so troubled that I cannot speak. I have considered the days of old, the year of ancient times. I call to remembrance my song in the night; I meditate within my heart, and my spirit makes diligent search. Will the Lord cast off forever? And will He be favorable no more? Has His mercy ceased forever? Has His promise failed forevermore? Has God forgotten to be gracious? Has He in anger shut up His tender mercies? Selah And I said, 'This is my anguish; **But** I will remember the years of the right hand of the Most High.' I will remember the works of the Lord; surely I will remember Your wonders of old. I will also meditate on all Your work, and talk of Your deeds. Your way, O God, is in the sanctuary; who is so great a God as our God? You are the God who does wonders; You have declared Your strength among the peoples." (Psalm 77:1-14)
- "For my soul is full of trouble, and my life draws near to the grave. I am counted with those who go down to the pit; I am like a man who has no strength,

   But to You I have cried out, O Lord, and in the morning my prayer comes before You." (Psalm 88:3-4, 13)
- "My heart is stricken and withered like grass, so that I forget to eat my bread. Because of the sound of my groaning my bones cling to my skin. My enemies reproach me all day long, and those who deride me swear an oath against me. My days are like a shadow that lengthens, and I wither away like grass. **But** You, O Lord, shall endure forever, and the remembrance of Your name to all generations." (Psalm 102:4-5, 8, 11-12)

- "My soul faints for Your salvation, **But** I hope in Your word." (Psalm 119:81)
- "Our bones are scattered at the mouth of the grave, as when one plows and breaks up the earth.

    But my eyes are upon You, O God the Lord; in You I take refuge; do not leave my soul destitute." (Psalm 141:7-8)

It's only by focusing on Him that we are able to list our blessings. We can have an attitude of gratitude in the midst of MS. Make a conscious effort to list your blessings when you are faced with more bad news. For me, my list included thanks: that God is real and more powerful than the disease, for the functions I still had (I thank the Lord each time I go to the bathroom because I know that, for some, incontinence is a symptom of the disease.), for promises in God's Word, that I was diagnosed (and not still left wondering what's wrong with me), that there are more and more treatments available, for family and friends, for the National MS Society, and that I'm the one who has the disease and not a loved one.

6) *Remember that He can help you keep a joyful spirit.* The Bible tells us that a merry heart doeth good like medicine (Proverbs 15:13). Intercessory prayers of faithful prayer warriors help me have a joyful countenance.

7) *Remember that His peace can replace anxiety.* Fear need not overtake us. In John 14:27 we read Jesus' own words saying, "'Peace I leave you, My peace I give to you; not as the world gives do I give to you. Let not your heart be troubled, neither let it be afraid.'" Because MS can affect any function at any time, fear is a reasonable response. When anxious thoughts begin to cross my mind, I like to read scripture, list my blessings, or listen to worship songs. That helps shift my focus. MS seems to take over the lives of those stricken with it.

I never forget, however, that there is always the possibility that my MS will affect my emotions or cognitive abilities. That's one reason I'm writing this book at this time. Currently, I am experiencing minor symptoms of a relapse. My hands are weak and I don't know if I will get paresthesia again (the painful pins and needles sensation in my hands that prevented me from typing once before). I live my life doing what I can while I still can. But looking to God helps me remember He is able. Therefore, I can live without fear. He is in control.

8) *Look to God for heavenly wisdom.* There is a lot of information to be found about MS if you look for it. Sometimes advice is shared with me unsolicited. It certainly is recommended that you learn all you can about MS. But it's important to learn the accurate and up to date facts. The National MS Society is the best source of information. Local chapters usually sponsor and advertise workshops so you can learn more about your disease. Register with your local chapter. Your neurologist will also be a good source of information since s/he knows the specific course of your illness and understands the disease. Be cautioned, however, when well-meaning friends share advice. For example I learned that since people with MS have an overactive immune system, taking some supplements that stimulate the immune system would be a bad thing to do. In addition people advised me to exercise (which is usually good advice for anyone), but my neurologist and physician were advising me not to exercise during a relapse (since I was too weak from my exacerbation). They told me that I would be referred at a later date to a physical therapist who would teach me how to do exercises properly. Simply starting exercises could be counterproductive to my well being. My neurologist once told me that undue stress during my exacerbation could weaken me further. Even when MS patients are not having a relapse it can take up to an hour to recover from exercise. But my neurologist also told me that he recommends that his MS patients remain as active as possible. I'm not opposed to exercising. In fact, I'm eager to be given the go ahead from my doctors. Exercising, eating properly, and getting sufficient sleep and rest is wise advice for anyone.

People with MS have to make many decisions. You have to select a neurologist. You have to determine which course of treatment you will use. Should you alter your plans (school, career, vacation, etc.)? Is it wise to tell your employer? You don't know whether or not you should get pregnant. In addition, you face the daily decisions of how much to push yourself. The one decision that should be clear in the life of a Christian is to commit all your actions to prayer, asking for the Lord to grant wisdom. He will direct your thoughts and give you direction.

Often the Lord uses family members and close friends to provide wisdom that you should follow. Obviously, the most important advice to heed (about your health decisions) is the advice given by your neurologist. Guard against trusting all the advice that comes your way. The Lord will make it clear which advice is from Him. He provides confirmations though several sources (especially through your neurologist).

9) *Remember that you are fearfully and wonderfully made.* God has created our bodies wonderfully in many ways (physically and emotionally). "I will praise You, for I am fearfully and wonderfully made . . ." (Psalm 139:14a) We were created with tear ducts. Even Jesus wept. In Ecclesiastes we read that there is, "A time to weep and a time to laugh; a time to mourn and a time to dance." (Ecclesiastes 3:4) Hearing sad news, such as the news that you have MS, makes us cry. There are many losses over the

course of a lifetime with MS. Losses lead to grief. Each time the disease takes a new course, especially at an extremely critical time in your life, crying is a natural response. However, wallowing in self pity is not healthy.

Our brain was also created wonderfully. The central nervous system (CNS) can repair itself. The National MS Society's booklet *Research Directions in Multiple Sclerosis* includes some encouraging new findings: "For decades it was believed that once myelin was lost in the CNS, it could not be regenerated. We now know that this is not true: The CNS can repair itself, or remyelinate . . . . The problem in MS seems to be that Myelin loss proceeds more aggressively and quickly than remelination. Understanding the myelination process is thus a vital area of research." There is hope in God's creation—this body we're stuck in. The Great Physician is leading researchers and scientists all around the world to new discoveries and treatments for MS. We can pray for a cure. One recent report found in the March 3rd, 2004 issue of USA Today related the results of an FDA approved study done at Hahnemann University Hospital in Philadelphia, PA. It stated, "Doctors report promising results using huge doses of a potent chemotherapy drug to treat autoimmune diseases including multiple sclerosis, though only a handful of patients have been treated so far and one MS researcher said far more study is needed before any victory is declared. The drug, cyclophosphamide, is given at such high doses that it destroys most or all of a patient's disease fighting immune cells. However, the stem cells within the patient's bone marrow survive the drug's onslaught, the doctors say, and then are stimulated with other drugs to rebuild the immune system from scratch—but without the bad triggers that caused the body to attack its own cells . . . Autoimmune diseases typically are suppressed with drug interferon, steroids, radiation, and other chemo drugs that stop reproduction of the confused cells that treat the body's own cells like they're foreign invaders. Brodsky's work involves killing the misdirected immune cells, not merely suppressing them . . . several of his patients who had cognitive problems, difficulty walking, or other coordination troubles have seen much of their symptoms disappear in as little as three to six weeks . . ." It was an amazing thing to learn that our stem cells can be stimulated to rebuild a new immune system from scratch. Our bodies are certainly fearfully and wonderfully made.

10) *Look unto heaven for the hope of new bodies.* "And God will wipe away every tear from their eyes; there shall be no more death, nor sorrow, nor crying; and there shall be no more pain, for the former things have passed away." (Revelation 21:4) There is great comfort in the knowledge that there will be a glorious time that we will no longer suffer any pain or sorrow. It helps to keep our focus on heaven. "For our citizenship is in heaven, from which we also eagerly wait for the Savior, the Lord Jesus Christ, who will transform our lowly body that it may be conformed to His glorious body, according to the working by which He is able even to subdue all things to Himself." (Philippians 3:20-21)

11) *Remember there is One who understands.* Many people with MS don't look like they have a disease. You can't really see or measure fatigue, pain, or depression. It's frustrating at times because no one seems to understand. But there is someone who knows our every thought and who understands. Reaching out to Him in prayer or by reading His Word provides the assurance that He knows what you're going through. Jesus tells us, "Come to Me, all you who labor and are heavy laden, and I will give you rest." (Matthew 11:28) He knows our frame and our frailties. That's why there is so much in the Bible about strength (literal and figurative). Refer to the chapter containing verses to find a list of verses on strength.

12) *Be prepared to yield yourself to a loving God.* Many people with MS find that they have to adjust their expectations, plans, and even goals. This can be very upsetting and discouraging unless you know that God has a perfect plan for your life. He holds your future. It is difficult to adjust to a change in plans. But it's easier to accept God's plan the more we understand His love for us. Daniel's three friends understood they served a loving God. When they faced being thrown into the furnace for refusing to worship any god except their own God, they said, ". . . our God whom we serve is able to deliver us . . . but if not . . ." (Daniel 3:17-18) They were willing to yield their bodies and worship God. That passage challenged me because I realized that God might have a higher purpose for me having MS. In the story with Daniel's friends, their commitment to God even got a Nebuchadnezzar's attention. He said God's angel "delivered His servants who trusted in Him . . . and yielded their bodies, that they should not serve nor worship any god except their own God'" (Daniel 3:28) We are assured of God's loving plans for us in Jeremiah. "For I know the thoughts that I think toward you, says the Lord, thoughts of peace and not of evil, to give you a future and a hope. Then you will call upon Me and go and pray to Me, and I will listen to you. And you will seek Me and find Me, when you search for Me with all your heart." (Jeremiah 29:11-13)

13) *Keep a journal to document God's provision.* Many people with MS keep a journal to keep track of their symptoms. This provides helpful information for your neurologist. Keeping a journal of how God has worked in your situation is helpful to you. Too often we forget about God's faithfulness. Even God's people forgot the miracles He performed for them. It seems hard to believe that they could complain because they didn't have water or food in the wilderness. How could they not know that the God who led them out of bondage and who opened the Red Sea would certainly provide food and water for them? If we have a record of what God has done, we can read it in times of discouragement. That can be a tool used to renew our hope.

The National MS Society acknowledges the value of spiritual beliefs. In their booklet *Multiple Sclerosis and Your Emotions* they recommend, "Faith is a very important part of most people's lives. Studies of people with chronic illness find that those who had a strong religious or philosophical belief system did better than those without such a source of support." So here again is the prescription for hope and strength:

1) Hope in Him, not in statistics.
2) Remember that God is your source of hope and strength.
3) Remember that He is in control.
4) Remember that He is faithful.
5) Focus on Him primarily.
6) Remember that He can help you keep a joyful spirit.
7) Remember that His peace can replace anxiety.
8) Look to God for heavenly wisdom.
9) Remember that you are fearfully and wonderfully made.
10) Look unto heaven for the hope of new bodies.
11) Remember there is One who understands.
12) Be prepared to yield yourself to a loving God.
13) Keep a journal to document God's provision.

The Bible offers a guideline for living with affliction: ". . . rejoicing in hope, patient in tribulation, continuing steadfastly in prayer;" (Romans 12:12) We can rejoice in hope and be patient in our tribulation if we continue steadfastly in prayer. We can find rest in hope. "I will bless the Lord who has given me counsel; my heart also instructs me in the night seasons. I have set the Lord always before me; because He is at my right hand I shall not be moved. Therefore my heart is glad, and my glory rejoices; my flesh also will rest in hope." (Psalm 16:7-9)

Chapter 2

Something is Wrong

On November 1, 2003 we were visiting our youngest son, Robert (21 years old) who was away at college. I noticed that my arms, legs, and abdomen were tingly. Since I had a cold at the time, I thought that the strange sensation was some sort of side effect of the cold.

But after two weeks it didn't go away. So, I went to my doctor, Dr. Kipp, who prescribed a battery of blood tests.

Shortly after, we learned that I did not have a thyroid problem, diabetes, or Lymes disease. So Dr. Kipp prescribed an MRI of my brain. On November 29th I had the MRI done. By then my hands were also tingly and very weak. I was told that I had paresthesia in my hands. They felt like I had on tight gloves lined with sand paper.

When I went to a follow up appointment with my doctor, he told me that he wanted to refer me to a neurologist who specializes in MS. He explained that the results of my MRI revealed that mylen was possibly damaged. Although I previously worked with someone who had MS, I didn't know what mylen was. He explained that it is kind of like the insulation of the nerve cells in my brain. I asked where in my brain the mylen was damaged. He told that he didn't see the actual MRI films; he only received the report. I asked to see the report. Before he showed me the report, he explained that damaged nerve cells show up as white spots on an MRI. When I attempted to read the report, I realized that it was written in a technical language I didn't really understand. However, there was one sentence that was frighteningly clear. It said that the white spots were "too numerous to count."

My masters in special education afforded me some understanding of the seriousness of my situation. Depending on the locations of white spots (which represented lesions in the brain), different functions could be affected (sight, speech, mobility, bladder control, emotions, cognitive functions, etc.).

Dr. Kipp, who attended my church and shared my faith, studied me as I read the report with an expression on his face that looked as if he was bracing for my reaction. I asked, "Do people fall apart when you tell them they have MS?" He answered compassionately, "Oh, yes." I suppose I didn't fall apart because I was thankful that, for a change, it wasn't my oldest son, Chris, who had the health problem. Chris was 23 years old and in his last year of college. When he was in elementary school he struggled with Attention Deficit Hyperactivity Disorder (ADHD). Then, in his junior year of high school, he had a psychotic episode and was diagnosed with schizoaffective disorder. That experience took me to new levels of dependence on the Lord. Later, he went on a church youth retreat and broke a rib while he had bronchitis. In his second year of college we learned that he has psoriatic arthritis which made every joint in his body stiff and sore. In his third year of college he had two severely herniated discs in his back. He found no relief after trying epidural shots. So he had back surgery. Even the removal of wisdom teeth wasn't routine for Chris; he hemorrhaged. So, I was thankful that he was not the one diagnosed with MS. (Chapter 8 has more details of his story. Or read my other book entitled *Journey From Insanity To Sanity; A Mother's Journey With Her Son.*

I was not able to get an appointment to see a local specialist until January 2, 2004. At the time I was teaching second grade. I managed to deal with my parasthesia by having the students help each other with zippers and opening things, since my hands didn't work well. But by December 8th I was so weak that when I arrived at work I was exhausted. Dr. Kipp advised me to go home since I was obviously unable to perform my duties. That was devastating news. The reality of my fatigue led me to tears. It was one thing to accept that I might have MS, but it was another to accept that I couldn't be with my students.

January 2nd seemed like such a long time to wait for an appointment.

That meant that I wouldn't even have a diagnosis until then. So I wouldn't be able to get treatment for whatever was wrong. I knew that Dr. Kipp thought I might have MS, but I wondered if I experienced a stroke, gotten cancer, or had an aneurysm in my brain. I felt helpless, frustrated, and extremely weak. January 2nd seemed like an eternity away.

CHAPTER 3

MY DIAGNOSIS

Since I taught at a Christian school, I had access to an army of people who would pray for me. I asked them to pray that I would be seen by a neurologist sooner than January 2nd. When I explained my situation, I told them that my MRI was abnormal—saying, "There's a news flash! My brain isn't normal." One day I remembered to call Chris's neuropsychiatrist, Dr. Nelson. I was supposed to have called him sooner with an update on how Chris was doing, but my situation made me forget to call him. I explained my symptoms and told him that I was waiting to see a neurologist who specializes in MS. With urgency in his voice, he told me that it's not good to wait. He urged me to begin calling specialists and get put on many waiting lists. That would increase the chances that an appointment would become available sooner. Suddenly I had renewed hope. I felt empowered. I began calling doctors immediately on a Friday. When I called Mt. Sinai Hospital in New York City, I was told an appointment was available that Monday (the very next work day)! I was beginning to see the Lord working mightily in my life.

Rob, who was a neuroscience major in college at the time, was home for his Christmas break. This provided him an opportunity to visit a doctor who specializes in MS. I told him not every mother would go to such extremes to provide a field trip for her son. Chris was also home from college. He stayed home with our two dogs. At Mt. Sinai's Corinne Goldsmith Dickinson Center for Multiple Sclerosis Dr. Tullman diagnosed me as having relapsing-remitting MS. In his report he stated, "Mrs. Chandler most surely has multiple sclerosis." He prescribed a course of high dose intravenous steroids (knowing that Dr. Kipp had already taken the usual first step by prescribing oral steroids). He also recommended that I begin treatment with a high dose of Rebif (one of the interferons, a disease modifying drug). He told me that whenever he puts patients on high dose IV steroids he usually hospitalizes them for observation. But since we didn't live in the New York City area, he told me that I would have to find a neurologist in my area who could monitor me while on the steroids.

On the way home in the car I made a phone call to a local neurologist that two people had recommended. Amazingly, an appointment was available the very next day. God is awesome! I would have a confirmation of the diagnosis and a second opinion the next day. I saw it as a blessing because many people are not so fortunate. They go many years before their MS is diagnosed. Since my blood tests all came back negative, and since my MRI revealed so many lesions, it was easier to make a diagnosis. A spinal tap wasn't even necessary.

When we returned home I told Chris that I do, in fact, have MS. Without missing a beat he responded, "Well at least you don't have PMS!" I was glad that he could keep his sense of humor in the situation. I told him that the neurologist prescribed IV steroids. I laid down to rest. The trip used up all the energy I had left. Chris came into my bedroom and sat down. He told me that he had just gone on the internet to find out more about steroids. His way of helping me was to provide me with information. He proceeded to list all the awful side effects of the medicine. As I lay listless in my bed listening to his report, I asked, "Is this my bedtime story? Does it have a happy ending?" The mood, thankfully, was light, yet serious.

The next day I met Dr. Mazlin, my neurologist. He concurred with Dr. Tullman. He agreed with the diagnosis of MS. He also agreed with the course of action: a high dose of IV Steroids and a high dose of Rebif. He also prescribed another MRI of my brain (with contrast this time) and an MRI of my cervical area. I didn't mind that because I welcome lying in the machine to get rest. I can even fall asleep during the procedure. He also prescribed an evoked potentials test (that measures the response of my CNS to specific stimulation). He said to me, "Since you're not acute I won't hospitalize you." I refrained from interjecting some humor and didn't say, "Hey, I think I'm pretty cute!" He explained that a nurse would visit my home to set me up with the IV steroids. I wouldn't have to be hospitalized. Both neurologists, however, were surprised that I wasn't having a more severe relapse given the numerous lesions on my brain. God's protection was evident.

All this was happening during the weeks leading up to Christmas. At school the students were rehearsing for their Christmas program. At home Rob was baking all the Christmas cookies. For decades I baked cookies for the family. I usually baked about 30-40 dozen cookies. This was a tradition I began even before I was married or had children. So when I had children they grew up helping me. Rob was quite able to bake them on his own, but I sat with him to join in on the joyous festivities. Although he was doing all the work, we still enjoyed each other's company. Rob was also making the dinner meals. Chris helped me before Rob came home for break, so Chris welcomed Robert's assistance. Robert also drove me to my appointments. Since I couldn't write well (due to the paresthesia), he filled out forms for me and took notes so I would remember what the doctor said. He had a willing spirit and seemed to be handling it all.

My husband, Howie, was helping with all the Christmas wrapping. He drove me to buy the remaining gifts for the boys. I was so weak that I became tired just walking into each store (even though Howie dropped me off at the door). Howie also came with me to the Christmas program at my school. I usually make a video of the entire year for my students' parents. The Christmas program had to be a part of the video tape, but I was too weak to do the taping. Howie agreed to help. As I waited for each of the younger grades to complete their part of the program, I felt weak and light-headed. I commented to Howie that I didn't know if I had enough energy to walk my students toward the platform. I told him that I was afraid I might pass out. In the Chandler style of coping, he asked, "Do you want me to film that? Here's Mrs. Chandler falling down." On the way out of school that night Howie checked the camcorder to see how much film and power remained. He said, "You have about an hour of energy left." I responded, "Well, I don't have an hour of energy left. It's pretty bad when I'm jealous of my camcorder!"

I had to explain to my students why I wasn't able to be at school. The principal sent home a letter to inform the parents that I had MS. She left it up to the parents to decide what and how much to tell their children. But I felt like I had to tell the students something. Many of them were concerned. So when I visited them for their Christmas party I explained that I feel like a wet noodle. I asked, "Do you understand what I mean when I say, 'I feel like a wet noodle?'" One student answered and said, "Yes, you feel kind of floppy." "Yes. That's right. I feel kind of floppy. And I can't really teach if I feel floppy. You can pray that the doctors know how to get all my energy back. Has anyone ever felt floppy?" I knew that they would rise to the occasion and share all their stories, which would divert the conversation away from any more details. That explanation seemed to satisfy them and they knew how to pray. I missed them desperately. Not being able to go to school was the hardest part.

Christmas Eve service was special, as always. I was grateful to have both boys home from college and my mother with us in church. Since my hands were weak and felt bad, I didn't close them. I just kept my hands resting in my lap open with palms up. Chris looked over at me before the service began and imitated me. He pretended he was meditating, touched his fingers to his thumbs with his palms up and said, "Urnmmm, uumm . . . ." I appreciated his dry sense of humor. I knew that he was filled with compassion for me. He, of all people, knew about pain and discomfort. At one time he gave me this advice: "Just because you have a pain doesn't mean you have to be one." He was a good example to me.

With all he's been through he doesn't have a complaining spirit. He is even thankful for his life. He's blessed in the knowledge that we love him unconditionally. We had to prove it to him when he assaulted us during a psychotic episode. He was not in his right mind and needed to be hospitalized. We visited him every day. Today, he is able to praise God no matter what. God blesses truth when you invested it in your children. In every difficult situation, we always told him that God has a reason for the trials in our lives—that He is working his perfect plan. You can trust God even when you can't track Him.

CHAPTER 4

IV STEROIDS

The IV steroids were an adventure right from the start. When the nurse came to the house Rob was busy baking cookies. She asked where I'd like for her to put the needle in my hand. I told her the kitchen had the best light. When she inserted the needle I got a vagal response. I felt the color go out of my face and I got light-headed. Right after than I began to feel nauseous. I asked to go lie down and the nurse wouldn't let me until she was sure that I wouldn't pass out. When she told me to just breathe I realized that I couldn't even breathe! As quickly as it all happened, it quickly went away. I felt better and could lie down. The nurse explained that the steroids need to be administered by hooking up a bag every six hours (at 6:00 AM, at noon, at 6:00 PM, and then at midnight). I asked how that worked. Would she come to the house for all those treatments for four days? She told me that someone would have to do it for me; they don't send nurses to administer each dose. I looked at Rob and said simply, "Rob? . . . ." He was happy to do it for me. I could trust him because he had performed surgery on rats. Although I wasn't a rat, I needed someone to do it and he was available and had something close to experience. So the nurse showed Rob how to hook up the bag and connect it to the needle in my hand.

When Rob approached me to administer the first dose on his own, I noticed that he had to disconnect a plastic lid to the Solu-Medrol—the clear steroid medicine that was in the bag. He did it in order to connect the tubing that would carry it into my vein. I stopped him and teasingly said, "Wait, do you have any unresolved issues with me?"

I was amazed at how much care and skill Rob used in giving me the doses. There was a time that the liquid wasn't flowing. Rob realized that the bag had to be higher in order for gravity to help it drip. Since I was lying down on my bed, Rob decided to hang the steroid bag from the ceiling fan. He jokingly threatened to turn on the fan.

The steroids really cut into Rob's sleep schedule. So Howie offered to do the midnight and 6:00 AM doses to give Rob a break. When Howie came to do his first dose, he walked up to the side of the bed and said, "Hi. I'm Howie and I'll be your doctor today. Let's pray." I remarked, "Wow, the other doctor never prayed with me. Maybe he's not a Christian." Of course Rob is a Christian.

That's evident in his gentleness and his servant heart. The humor broke the tension.

The steroids also interfered with my sleep. They prevented me from sleeping soundly. Usually I only got three or four hours of sleep each night while on the IV steroids. That afforded me lots of quiet time to read the Bible and pray. That's when I began my own study on strength. I found that the Bible has a great deal to say about strength. I also found renewed hope. God promises to provide physical and inner strength. Reading all the passages about affliction provided the encouragement and comfort I needed.

The mother of one of my students was a nurse. She warned me that steroids can really mess with someone's emotions especially when you are weaned off them. After four days with the IV steroids, I was scheduled for 12 days of oral steroids (with gradually decreasing doses). It was referred to as a 12 day taper, but Howie called it my 12 days of Christmas. I already knew about the possible effect on emotions because Chris had researched it on the internet and shared it with me. But I told Robert that I might be a little emotional as I go off the steroids; I might not act normal. He said, "Why is this news?" I really didn't mind his response because I work hard at not being normal. Later another parent of one of my students shared her personal experience with steroids and how they made her very emotional. So, I warned Chris. He said, "That's OK, Mom. We'll just lock you in your room 'till it's all over." I told him he might hear me calling from my room, "Steroids! Steroids! I need my steroids!" Happily for all, I didn't experience any extreme emotions (as far as I know!).

I don't really know if the steroids shortened my relapse. When school resumed after the holidays I was still very weak. Both my neurologist and my physician told me they didn't think I was ready to return to work. That was hard for me to accept. Dr. Mazlin told me that I could probably go back to work as long as they knew I'd need help. Fortunately, the headmaster assured me he would have a substitute in with me as long as I needed it. He added that we could take it one day at a time. I felt so blessed to have that kind of support from my employer.

I also felt unbelievably blessed by the outpouring of love, prayers, and offers to help. One dear friend of mine had recently had back surgery. When she learned about my diagnosis she called me. She offered to provide a meal for my family. I asked, "How are you going to do that? You're recovering from surgery." She told me that she planned on mailing me a ham and turkey. That taught me an important lesson. Anyone can find a way to serve the Lord. It also convicted me to keep my eyes off myself during my illness and look for others who might need a touch of God's love. It was hard for me to be on the receiving end of kindness. But I learned that with MS I need to accept help. MS can certainly cause an adjustment in self image. I needed to alter my assessment of my abilities. I was accustomed to doing everything myself. Now, I had to get used to needing help at times. But I needed to remind myself that God has a purpose for all He allows. For example, Howie was always more tender to me when I was sick. When I got meningitis or when I suffered a back injury he was very helpful and compassionate. He's used to seeing me as a strong pillar. But when I'm sick he's very attentive. That's a good thing for our marriage.

I also got to see my mother more often when I was extremely weak or getting steroids. She'd drive one hour from her house to come and clean for me, make dinner, and drive me places. Chris asked, "What would motivate a woman her age to drive one hour and clean three bathrooms?" I responded, "-the love of a mother." My mom often brought me gifts that were extremely thoughtful—gifts that only a mother would know to give. She brought me some mittens because she knew that wearing gloves would be uncomfortable with my paresthesia. My hand would hurt even if Howie held my hand. She also bought me a loose fitting sweater that would easily fit over my hand while I was getting my IV steroid treatments. We had more opportunities for fellowship than our busy schedules would normally allow.

CHAPTER 5

MY RESPONSE AND REACTIONS FROM OTHERS

My initial reaction to learning I have MS was mixed feelings. I was mostly relieved. For a long time I knew that something was wrong with me since I was always so tired. Now I knew that I really was more tired than people who don't have MS. It wasn't my imagination. I also was relieved to find out that I wasn't simply out of shape and getting old. Somehow, for me, there was less shame in having MS than in being pathetically out of shape.

I was also amazed at God's provision and protection. The previous year I had a parent volunteer who helped me every Friday all day. That was in addition to another parent who helped me for two hours every Wednesday. Both parents realized that everyone got blessed by their help. They got to see and hear what happens in their child's day. Their children loved to have their mothers spend part of the day or the whole day with them in the classroom. All the other students enjoyed having another adult in the room to help them. And I certainly appreciated their help. So, at Back to School Night I did a little 'commercial' advertising the benefits of volunteering in the classroom. I was overwhelmed by the response! I got six parents who volunteered their time on a regular basis. Starting in September I trained those dear ladies to follow my method of grading the students' papers, to know where to find the list of what needed to be done, to know how to use the copy machine, etc. So, when I suddenly had to be out of school in December, the parent volunteers knew exactly what needed to be done. All I needed to do was to give them a quick phone call.

It was interesting to see how God prepared Robert's heart for this new adventure of mine. Prior to my diagnosis and even before I had gotten the first MRI of my brain, Robert did a report in college on multiple sclerosis. He could have chosen any topic but he chose MS. So when he heard the news that I have MS, he had some understanding of what that meant. He was able to share information with me that was helpful.

As I said before, I was thankful for God's protection. When I discovered that lesions had been forming in my brain for years, I was thankful that I hadn't had a severe relapse. I was grateful that I had been able to help start the school and that I was able to minister to Chris when he needed me.

But all my reactions weren't positive. I was frustrated about the interruption in my life. I quickly became impatient with the relapse. My neurologist, Dr. Mazlin, told me that if I did in fact have MS for a while, then the course of my disease had been mild. He told me the past course of the disease is a good predictor of how the disease will progress. So I expected to be done with my relapse and move on with life until the next relapse, which I didn't expect for a while.

What I've learned about MS is that "I don't know" is the standard answer from doctors. Since the disease takes a different path in every individual, doctors can't predict how MS will impact patients. Although there is quite a bit of research going on about MS and new treatments are being developed every day, there is still a lot that is not known. When we went to Mt. Sinai Hospital in New York City, I was telling Dr. Tillman about my symptoms. When I told him about the paresthesia, I asked if it would go away. He answered solemnly, "I don't know." I'm sure he would have liked to assure me that it would go away. The fact is that some symptoms during a relapse remain after the relapse is over. Later in the car going home, I reminded Rob of that response and teasingly said, "See, Rob. He went to medical school to learn how to say, 'I don't know'."

Doctors don't know how long a relapse will take (from a few days to six months). The first two people I spoke to who had MS both had a relapse that lasted six months. So I declared, "That's just not going to happen with me. That would keep me out of school for the rest of the year. I'm done with it now!" I knew that my words wouldn't magically make it so, but it felt good pretending that I had some kind of control.

So I explained my plans to Dr. Mazlin who didn't really know me yet. I told him that I needed to be back to work. I told him that there were 21 little second graders who were praying that I'd return to school. I asked him what he could do to help me meet my goal to return to work after Christmas vacation. Besides recommending that I get assistance, he gave me samples of medication to give me energy (Provigil).

When I visited my primary physician, Dr. Kipp, for a follow up appointment I reported to him about my visit to Dr. Mazlin. He commented on how I seemed better. Since I didn't have any make-up on and I still felt extremely weak, I asked him why he made that statement. Since he knew me better than Dr. Mazlin, he knew that as long as I have a plan I'm happy. I had a plan to return to work—with help. When I told him that Dr.

Mazlin gave me medication to increase my energy level, he slowly nodded his head and said, "I'm going to have to speak to that man." He's gotten to know that I'm happier when I'm busier. Although he knew that I was weak, he couldn't imagine me with more energy than I usually have. What would that be like?!

After I was first diagnosed, each day was a new adventure with my body. New symptoms were always showing up and I didn't know what was related to the MS, what was related to medication, or what was not really noteworthy. For example, I began getting headaches. I didn't know if it was from the steroids or lack of sleep. The steroids prevented me from sleeping much. Perhaps it was a symptom of the relapse. Dr. Mazlin believed that it was from the Provigil. He told me to stop taking it. I didn't get another headache. That was sort of a good thing because Provigil is extremely expensive if managed health plans don't approve it. But I was also sad to give up the Provigil. It was my only hope for strength. Now I had to rely on answered prayers for restored energy. So the Lord got me back to the place where my total trust had to be in Him.

Trusting God is easier said than done. I think it somehow helps when you understand more of His character. So often when we pray and still struggle with life, we assume that we didn't pray correctly or that God didn't hear. It helps me to think of how much I love my own sons and what I'd do for them. If they were in danger, my care and protection wouldn't depend on how (of if) they asked for help. I wouldn't hesitate to assist them. But my powers are limited.

If I reflect on my sons' physical power, I feel comfortable with their ability to protect me. Rob and Chris both have their black belts in karate. Chris continues to lift weights. Rob used to wrestle in high school. In college he worked toward his second black belt in another form of martial arts. When I go somewhere with them especially at night I feel very secure and safe. I'm confident that if any danger faced us they would be completely capable of protecting me. I wouldn't have to ask for their protection because I know they love me.

That's the way it is with God. He loves us so much that He will protect us even if we don't use what we think are all the right words when we speak to Him in prayer. However He tells us to present our requests to Him so that when He reveals His answer, we realize that the answer came from Him. We then recognize that God met a need. God can solve our problems if we rely on Him instead of on our own abilities or intellect. Sadly, at times I've asked God for His help and preceded to solve my own problems. Our understanding of what He can do is so limited that we hold on to our fears. His power is limitless. He is able to care for us beyond our imagination. It is His pleasure to reveal His power and love for us in response to our specific requests.

When I reflected on the timing of my relapse, I realized that God's timing is always perfect. Both boys were home for Christmas. So, they were able to see how I was doing first hand. They were able to help me. I couldn't imagine them away at school hearing about what was going on and not being able to see me or to help. They might have imagined that I was worse than I really sounded over the phone. This way, they could know for sure that I was doing well—being covered in the prayers of others and supported with help from everyone. It wasn't until Chris was back at school (in April) that he had a hard time dealing with me having MS.

My other response was to find out all I could about my disease and at the same time not let MS take over our lives. I was determined to have everyone in the family go on with their lives. I was determined to keep all our family holiday traditions. That may not be realistic thinking for a person with MS who has debilitating side effects. Fortunately, I had done much of my Christmas shopping in the summer and fall. We were able to do much of what we normally do working as a team. For example, we always have a Christmas Eve dinner at our house with my mother and aunt attending. It was important to me to keep that special tradition. It always marked the end of all the secular details associated with Christmas and the beginning of a real focus on Jesus coming to earth as a babe. Howie, Chris, and Robert did just about all of the work under my direction. I really resisted helping because I just dropped things. In addition, running my hands under water was painful. So I was thankful for their help. It was a Christmas Eve dinner that I'll cherish.

Around that time I was getting phone calls from relatives who heard the news that I have MS. My brother, Ken, called me. He told me about a conversation that he had with Robert. Ken was asking Robert about his music. Robert was a music minor in college. He's got quite a gift for music. In high school he entered competitions and won a place in the county band, the district band, and the regional band. In addition, he was chosen to be one of the two drum majors of his marching band. While being a drum major, he won the award for 'Best Drum Major' at two different competitions.

Actually, Rob's not the only family member with a gift for music. Howie took piano lessons for 10 years while growing up. He can hear a song he doesn't know and instantly play it on the piano. He could then immediately transpose it to another key if it was too high for a singer. Chris, too, has a musical gift. He also won positions in the county and district bands. He also auditioned for a spot in Penn State's Marching Blue Band and was chosen. He played in their marching band for two years (one with two herniated discs and one after back surgery). I, on the other hand, have no musical talent at all. I took five long years of piano as a child. That was enough to appreciate real talent. So Ken was interested in one of Robert's passions—music. Ken asked Rob, "What's the hardest thing for you at your level?" Robert told him, "The rests." You need to pay attention to the rests so that you don't come in at the wrong time. Since Robert played the trombone, it wouldn't be a good thing to come in at the wrong time. Ken related that part of the conversation to me and then added, "So, Vic, take care of your rests." He knew that it would be hard for me to stop and rest. But he knew that it would be important for me to take care of my body. I was blessed by his concern.

My sister's advice was very direct, as usual. Like me, she used to be a special education teacher. Special ed. teachers have to know how to be very compassionate and also very direct. She has the perfect temperament for that. She knows how to handle me with care and understanding, looking out for my interests. She knows that I'm usually too busy looking out the interests of others. That's the way it is with most moms. She told me to keep in mind that I can apply for Social Security Disability benefits if that becomes necessary. She offered to help me since that's her line of business. I was thankful that I had a sister like Peggy.

Whenever I dropped things because of the weakness in my hands, I thought back to the first students that I had. I began my career as a special ed. teacher. I taught multi handicapped students. They were all legally blind. In addition they were all mildly retarded. Some of them had difficulty walking or were in wheelchairs. Most of them struggled with emotional problems as a result of their disabilities and limited understanding of their situations. However, many of them maintained a healthy sense of humor. Suddenly I felt a bond with them even though it had been 25 years since I taught them. The memory of their response to life was an inspiration to me.

My father was also an example to me. The way he dealt with lung cancer taught me how to live with pain and discomfort. Although he'd been gone for over ten years, I still remembered his last days in the hospital. With his last breath he thought of everyone else. He did his taxes and gave wise advice to everyone. He showed me that it's possible to think of others in the midst of pain. I'm thankful for such a strong heritage.

My response to the diagnosis of MS and its symptoms was shaped, in part, by how my loved ones responded. Their supportive words, prayers, and help eased my burden. Their humor lifted me up. You can't control the disease, but with God's help you can control your response to the disease.

CHAPTER 6

BLOTCHES AND BRUISES

Some have tried to comfort me by saying, "If you have to be diagnosed with MS, now is a good time. Just ten years ago, there was little that doctors could do to treat the disease. Now there are relatively new FDA approved drugs to control the disease and there are drugs to alleviate the symptoms." When someone first shared that line of comfort my first thought wasn't, "Yippee! Now I'm so happy to have MS." I was still unhappy to have the disease. But then I thought about those individuals who were diagnosed decades ago and who are wheelchair bound or who can't talk or who can't see. Then those words were a gentle reminder to me that I am fortunate. With a disease like MS you have to search for the hidden blessings. Doing that helps build a grateful spirit.

Although I continue to rely on the Lord for peace in my situation, it's still no fun. If I didn't acknowledge the discomfort and sadness, I'd be in denial. It's important to admit honest thoughts and feelings. I don't like my treatment. The treatment that both neurologists recommended in my case was high dose Rebif. It's a form of interferon that must be injected three days a week. It is a disease modifying drug. In the National MS Society's booklet *Plaintalk, A Booklet about MS for Families* they explain that interferons, "slow the rate of relapses, slow the onset of disability, and limit MS activity in the brain, as seen on MRI scans."

When I agreed to use the Rebif, my neurologist gave me a box to take home. It contained information about the drug. It even contained a video tape about the medication. What kind of medication comes with a movie? Since my hands felt like pins and needles and were extremely weak, Howie agreed to give me my injections. Together, he and I watched the video. It told us about studies that were done to prove the effectiveness of the medication. Although it had only recently been approved by the FDA in the United States, it had been used in Canada for a long time. So they had quite a bit of data to prove its effectiveness. The video also demonstrated the proper way to administer the shots.

It's safe to assume that most people don't like needles. I've even heard of some people with MS who are so squeamish that they can't take any interferon medicine at all (since they all have to be administered by injection). I happen to be included among those who'd rather not ever get another shot. But all of a sudden I was faced with the reality that this would be my life. I'd have to get three shots a week for the rest of my life or until a cure is found for the disease.

This presented another challenge for me to keep a sense of humor and to look to God instead of feeling sorry for myself. Whenever Chris had to face unpleasant things in his life I reminded him that there are people who face much greater challenges or much worse situations. We can just turn on the TV to see war in other countries. What kind of life must those people have? Certainly worse than mine. Other people live in poverty, live in dangerous neighborhoods, suffer oppression or continued abuse, face a lifetime of operations, or have a terminal illness. Thankfully MS isn't usually fatal. So I gave myself the same advice I'd given Chris so often. It did help me deal with it. Positive self talk can help shift your perspective. In the Bible we have Paul's example of keeping an eternal perspective in the midst of pain, persecution, and suffering. He was just a man and yet didn't wallow in self-pity. I marvel at his response in spite of what he went through. In II Corinthians we read Paul's own list of his suffering. ". . . in labors more abundant, in stripes above measure, in prisons more frequently, in deaths often. From the Jews five times I received forty stripes minus one. Three times I was beaten with rods; once I was stoned; three times I was shipwrecked; a night and a day I have been in the deep; in journeys often, in perils of waters, in perils of robbers, in perils of my own countrymen, in perils of the Gentiles, in perils in the city, in perils in the wilderness, in perils in the sea, in perils among false brethren; in weariness and toil, in sleeplessness often, in hunger and thirst, in fastings often, in cold and nakedness—besides the other things, what comes upon me daily: my deep concern for all the churches. Who is weak, and I am not weak?" (II Corinthians 11:23-29)

He wasn't happy with his situations. He didn't enjoy suffering. Later in II Corinthians we find out exactly how much he hated pain. "And lest I should be exalted above measure by the abundance of the revelations, a thorn in the flesh was given to me, a messenger of Satan to buffet me, lest I be exalted above measure. Concerning this thing I pleaded with the Lord three times that it might depart from me. And He said to me, 'My grace is sufficient for you, for my strength is made perfect in weakness.' Therefore most gladly I will rather boast in my infirmities, that the power of Christ may rest upon me. Therefore I take pleasure in infirmities, in reproaches, in needs, in persecutions, in distresses, for Christ's sake. For when I am weak, then I am strong." (II Corinthians 12:7-10)

Several things in that passage spoke to my heart. Paul pleaded for the 'thorn in the flesh' to depart. It's OK to take your honest requests to the Lord. Ask Him to remove the pain, the suffering, and the symptoms of the disease. I also realized that God could use the MS to do a work in my heart. Paul's comment, "lest I should be exalted above measure . . . a thorn in the flesh was given to me" indicates that Paul realized God was doing a work in his heart. I also was comforted by the reminder that God can be my strength. Paul recognized that he could gain strength from God. He said, "For when I am weak, then I am strong." (II Corinthians 12:10)

In Romans Paul lists all the work God does in the hearts of people facing trials. "And not only that, but we also glory in tribulations, knowing that tribulation produces perseverance; and perseverance, character, and character, hope. Now hope does not disappoint, because the love of God has been poured out in our hearts by the Holy Spirit who was given to us. For when we were still without strength, in due time Christ died for the ungodly." (Romans 5:3-6)

James, also, points out that God's purpose for trials is to do a work in our hearts. "My brethren, count it all joy when you fall into various trials, knowing that the testing of your faith produces patience." (James 1:2) Well, I don't know if I'm at a place where I count it all joy. However, it's a good start to understand that God has a loving purpose for my suffering.

It also helps to remember that God has other reasons for suffering. In II Corinthians we read, "Blessed be the God and Father of our Lord Jesus Christ, the Father of mercies and God of all comfort, who comforts us in all our tribulation, that we may be able to comfort those who are in any trouble, with the comfort with which we ourselves are comforted by God." (II Corinthians 1:3-4) As long as we live in this world we will have trials. The comfort we receive from the Lord and lessons we learn from Him can benefit others as we share with people in similar circumstances.

Dr. Mazlin prepared me for the possible side effects I might experience. He said that most people experience flu like symptoms. He added, "It's rare not to experience flu like symptoms. I don't know why some people don't get flu like symptoms." I read about all the other possible side effects. One of the bad side effects is depression or even thoughts of suicide. Great! The disease won't kill me but the medicine might cause me to do it myself. I sent out the word to all my faithful prayer warriors to pray that I don't get flu like symptoms or any other bad side effects.

A visiting nurse came to our house to get us started with the Rebif. He explained that the best way to give the injection is to pinch the skin with one hand and "shoot it like a dart" into the skin with the other hand and then slowly inject the medicine. Happily when Howie gave me my first injection there was no pain as he put the needle in like a dart. But there was a painful, burning sensation when he injected the medicine. I've since learned that there is a burning sensation because the injections come premixed.

Thankfully, I didn't experience any flu like symptoms from the Rebif. My students had been praying for me, asking God to keep me from feeling like I have the flu. It was nice for them to witness the answer to their prayers. When we first started with the Rebif injections Howie and I had some 'technical difficulties.' For example, several of the first few times Howie said, "The needle didn't go in. Your skin must be tough." I told him that couldn't be the reason, so we both carefully examined the needle. It looked sharp enough. I reminded him, "Just shoot it like a dart! Just jab that thing in me." It must be hard to give someone you love an injection. It wasn't easy for Howie to jab that sharp needle in me.

Eventually, he became more confident and has gotten quite skilled at shooting it like a dart into me.

Another complication that we encountered was when a needle broke, preventing Howie from getting it into my skin. Since I don't like to watch the needle going into me, Howie informed me, "The needle broke." I asked in shock, "What do you mean, 'The needle broke'?" He repeated, "The needle broke!" My cousin, Kate, who used to be an operating room nurse enjoyed hearing stories about our injection problems. We were such amateurs. One time when I got an injection the burning sensation was considerably worse and lasted for hours. There was a phone number that I could call and speak to a nurse who was familiar with people taking Rebif. I called that number and explained about the burning sensation that lasted so long. The nurse told me that the needle must have gone into a nerve. Yikes! No wonder it was so sore. The nurse reviewed with me where to do the injections. When I got the information about Rebif there was a picture of a person with rectangles in various spots indicating where the injections should be administered. My choices were: on the top of my thighs, on my buttocks, on my abdomen, or underneath my upper arms (on the part that wobbles if you haven't lifted weights lately— or ever!!!). Howie and I thought we had selected a recommend spot, but obviously the picture wasn't clear. What they should tell you is to stay far away from the crack in your butt! Since I teach at a Christian school the teachers and staff have morning devotions at 8:00 AM each day. On Wednesdays we break into smaller groups so people feel more free to share very personal prayer requests. The next day was Wednesday so I shared my news with the ladies. I said. "FYI: You might need to know this someday . . . If you're getting an injection in your butt, it's good to stay away from the crack!"

The very next time Howie gave me an injection, he was careful not to give me the injection in the wrong place. I told him what the nurse told me on the phone and we looked again at the picture of the person with rectangles. He said, "I have to find a spot with enough fat to pinch. OK, here's a spot with a lot of fat." I wasn't sure how to respond to that!!! It wasn't really an assessment of my figure. It was more of a comment to lovingly assure me that he found a good place to give me the injection.

On an earlier occasion I called the phone number to get advice from a nurse. The nurse gave me helpful information. She told me that other patients have experienced less burning when they take the needle out of the refrigerator in the morning instead of only 30 minutes before the injection is administered (My form of interferon has to be refrigerated since it's premixed.). They also told me that if I take Aleve at least 30 minutes before my injection I wouldn't experience any headaches or flu like symptoms. I learned, also, that many MS patients use cold compresses to ease the discomfort of the injection site. However, I shouldn't use them immediately after the injection is administered because I need to give the medication a chance to be absorbed into the skin. That was OK with me because I learned that after a brief burning sensation, there was a period when the injection site got numb and there was no pain at all. Then if there was going to be discomfort, I felt it later.

When I'd feel the burning sensation it helped me to thank the Lord for the medicine. I was truly thankful that there was something that would reduce the number of relapses I'd have and slow the onset of a disability. It seemed a small price to pay. I sometimes would think of my sister. She had recently been treated for breast cancer. Following her treatments for the cancer, she began the process to reconstruct her breasts. The doctors put a port in her chest so they could inject a saline solution. Each time she went for the injections they had difficulty locating her port. They would sometimes take up to 20 minutes trying to locate her port. I couldn't imagine the pain she endured. So, I was able to tolerate a few seconds of a burning sensation. I read the literature that accompanied the Rebif and realized they warned about possible 'injecton site reactions.' That was their way of describing blotches and bruises. I prefer to describe them as I see them.

Sometimes when Howie gave me the injection in my abdomen there would be a little bleeding. So, once again, I called the phone number to get advice. The nurse informed me that sometimes people hit a small corpuscle that causes the bleeding. She assured me that it wasn't a problem.

I also learned during that conversation that it's best to let the area that has been cleaned with alcohol dry completely to prevent any burning from the alcohol. I was getting to know that helpful phone number by heart.

The title of this chapter, 'Blotches and Bruises' was chosen because the blotches and bruises caused by the injections were my greatest challenge. When I first saw the blotches that were left at the injection sites, I thought we were doing something wrong. The lady in the Rebif video had perfectly clear skin on her thigh. I didn't recall reading or hearing about blotches. So I called the nurse for advice. She told me that the blotches were normal. Furthermore, they usually take up to three weeks to go away. She recommended that I try aloe gel on my skin to clear up the blotches faster. She even specified that I use the gel after I take my shower while my pores are open. Using the lotion would also have the benefit of preventing my skin from becoming leathery.

With three shots a week and each blotch taking up to three weeks to go away, it was getting increasingly more difficult to locate a good spot for my injections. Surely I didn't want to get an injection in an already irritated spot. I remember reading that some people keep a record of where and when each injection was given so they don't get an injection in a spot that was recently used. I couldn't understand why anyone would need to do that. All I had to do was to just look at my skin! If there was a blotch or a bruise I knew that it wasn't a good spot. My solution was to ask for prayer. I knew that the Lord is able to clear up those spots. I also knew that I'd get lots of advice about how to solve my problem. What I didn't expect was a gift I received from one teacher. She had recently traveled to Aruba. She gave me the Aloe gel she got from Aruba! I felt very blessed. I knew that if it worked I'd have to travel to Aruba to get more. Another lady at work offered to grow an Aloe plant for me.

My small group of ladies I prayed with on Wednesdays had a different response to my prayer request. At lunch on a Tuesday two of the ladies snickered when I walked into the room. When I asked them what they were up to, they told me they were planning on bringing markers to small group prayer the next day. They said they wanted to connect my dots!!! I suggested they bring a highlighter instead so they could highlight areas that were OK for Howie to use.

I couldn't even use all of the recommended areas. I found out the hard way that the injection sites were tender. I never paid attention to the fact that I closed the drawer of my desk at school with my thigh until I did it after an injection. I quietly said to myself, "OK, that hurt. I'll have to remember not to do that again." But I didn't remember. I still close that drawer with my thigh. Old habits never die. I also never paid attention to the fact that the counter in my classroom is as high as the top of my bottom. One day I leaned against the counter and felt pain. I never used to feel pain when I leaned. You're not supposed to feel pain when you lean back against something. This was a new and unpleasant sensation. Then I realized that I leaned against an injection site. I never used to pay attention to how far I pull my stockings down when I go to the bathroom. After I started using my thighs for injection sites you better believe I started paying attention to that. Nylon stockings can really jab into tender skin. But I figured out that if I didn't use the spot where I pull my stockings down to I'd be OK. I also learned to be careful in how I crossed my legs. If I crossed one leg over the other and rested it on my thigh that would cause discomfort. So I cross my legs behind one another at the calf. I understand that that's better for circulation anyway. In addition, it apparently looks more ladylike that way. That's how Princess Diana did it.

I also asked Dr. Kipp if he had any suggestions or solutions to my blotch problem. He gave me samples of Elidel. I didn't notice any improvement with that. It's still difficult to find good places to get my injections.

There was one time that I was able to laugh about it. Howie likes to approach me slowly and gently with the needle. By accident he said, "I'm going to punch you now—I mean pinch you." I told him, "No wonder I have bruises!!" It was so funny to me that I couldn't stop laughing. Howie couldn't give me the shot until I stopped laughing because my abdomen was moving. Maybe then he really thought about punching me!

Another time my injection resulted in a bruise the size of a tennis ball. It was located toward the inside of my thigh. Several doctors told me we had hit a corpuscle. I thought someone should develop a corpuscle finder—an instrument similar to a stud finder that would help you stay away from corpuscles.

CHAPTER 7

ACCEPTANCE (AN ONGOING PROCESS)

From the second week of January until the first week of March I felt better. I noticed that I didn't get my period for two months in a row. I knew that the Rebif could affect my menstrual period so I wasn't concerned. Dr. Mazlin confirmed that the Rebif was probably the cause of the change and wasn't concerned about it. My right leg and my right arm seemed very weak but that wasn't a big concern to me. I could deal with that. It was just hard to muster the energy to climb the five steps out of the building at the end of the day. But I figured it was just regular fatigue I'd have to deal with from my MS. I felt like I was finished with my relapse.

I seemed to have sufficient energy to teach without someone helping me. But my two grade level partners (the other two second grade teachers) watched my class at their lunch time so I'd have a longer rest in the middle of the day. They also walked my students out to recess. They were a tremendous source of support. The principal constantly checked on me to see if I was OK. She knew I didn't want to ask for help or complain about my symptoms, so she pointedly asked me, "How are you doing?"

The only two times I found that I was unusually exhausted were when we went on a field trip and when we started a new hot lunch procedure with the students. Field trips wear out all teachers. I certainly would get tired after a field trip, but after one night sleep I'd feel better. In February I was still exhausted three days after the field trip! That was discouraging. When we started the new hot lunch procedure (which required a lot of standing, walking around, and concentration) I was more exhausted than any other teacher. Just when I felt like I was finished with my relapse I'd have an experience like that.

In February I got information in the mail from the National MS Society informing me of two workshops in my area. One of the workshops was going to be held at a local restaurant and lunch would be provided for free. I told Howie, "Hey, there are perks to having MS. I get a free lunch! Do you wanna come with me?" He answered, "I'm not the one with MS."

But I reminded him that MS affects the whole family. I assured him that he'd get a free lunch too. Sure enough we attended the workshop, learned a lot from a local specialist, and had a wonderful meal. The meal was attended by many people in wheelchairs or using canes. I asked Howie if he was prepared to see that. He said that he expected to see some of that.

On Monday, March 8ᵐ I thought I had a slight dizzy spell at work. I chalked it up to a change in my sugar level. I was still learning what is associated with MS and what isn't. I didn't want to run to my doctor for every little thing. The next day I felt another dizzy spell. That night I was scheduled to see Dr. Kipp for a regular follow-up appointment. So I mentioned the dizzy spells to him. I also told him about the weakness in my right arm and leg. He asked me if I told my neurologist about those symptoms. I asked him, "What could he do about it anyway?" He answered, "He could put you on steroids again." So I planned on calling Dr. Mazlin the next day.

The next day, Wednesday, I woke up and realized that I was dizzy. It wasn't my imagination and it wasn't just a dizzy spell. The dizziness was constant. By the time I got to work it seemed as if it was quickly getting worse. I wondered if I would be OK to drive home. I knew that dizzy spells can be a signal of a relapse. When I called Dr. Mazlin he told me that he wanted me to begin another four days of IV steroids again. I was very upset. I had planned for my students to use the computer lab in the high school that Friday and didn't want to disappoint them. So I asked the principal if I could come in for that activity. She reminded me that after receiving IV steroids my immune system would be weakened for 18 months (which is what my doctor told me). With all the illness that was going around the school she knew I wouldn't want to get sick. Any illness hits a person with MS harder. So I had to cancel the computer lab activity.

I called Howie at work to tell him that I needed to get IV steroids again. He got off the phone and told his 'buddy' that I was dizzy. His friend shot back the comment, "They're ALL dizzy!"

The next day I knew I had made the right decision to stay home from work because I had become significantly weaker. My right arm and right leg were not only weak, but I felt a constant ache in my leg. I wondered if I was having another relapse or if it was the same relapse. I was bracing myself to hear more news I'd have to accept.

I didn't really pay attention to the pain and weakness in my leg because I was so concerned about my energy level in general. I could teach with pain and weakness in my arm and leg, but I couldn't teach without sufficient energy. I also didn't pay any attention to the pain and weakness in my leg when I had parasthesia because the weakness and discomfort in my hands significantly affected my daily activities. But when I thought about the pain in my leg I remembered that I had noticed the pain as far back as September of 2003. I started to wonder if I had secondary-progressive MS. With relapsing-remitting MS a person has a relapse (also called a flare or an exacerbation) which is followed by a period of recovery or remission (when symptoms go away completely or partially). But with secondary-progressive MS the person has attacks followed by partial recovery and their symptoms and disabilities slowly become worse. Currently there aren't many options available to slow the course of secondary-progressive MS. Some neurologists are prescribing Mitoxantrone that is a powerful immune suppressing medication. According to the National MS Society's *Living With MS* booklet, it is "a powerful immune suppressing medication with a limited life-time dosage to prevent heart damage." There are other medications being considered to treat the secondary-progressive form of MS. Among them are chemotherapy drugs used to treat cancer.

On my next visit with Dr. Mazlin I reminded him that Dr. Tullman (from Mt. Sinai Hospital in NYC) believed I might have a progressive form of the disease. I asked Dr. Mazlin if he thought I might have secondary-progressive MS. He thought it was too early to determine that.

On the day I felt the first dizzy spell (March 8ᵗʰ) our two cocker spaniels had an appointment to get shots at the vet. Our older dog, Zelda, who was 12 years old had some sort of growth on her hind leg that was about the size of a golf ball. I figured it was just a lump that she had due to her old age. Many dogs get lumps that are simply cysts—nothing to worry about. But when the vet saw it he informed us that, although she did not have cancer, the lump was a tumor. Left untreated, the tumor would grow quickly and eventually cause her pain and impair her ability to walk.

Upon hearing the news I began to cry. I told the vet that I was surprised at my reaction since I didn't even cry like that when I learned I had MS. The compassionate man explained that our dog meant a lot to everyone in the family. This news about her might upset my loved ones in the family. He didn't know how right he was. We originally got Zelda when Chris was in 5ᵐ grade to help him through a very difficult time in his life. Later when Chris was struggling with mental illness, Zelda was a tremendous source of comfort. This news would be hard to break to Chris. I could accept pain for myself better than sadness for my loved ones.

The vet said that since the tumor was already so large he wouldn't be able to remove it. He recommended another vet who might be able to remove it. I realized that difficult surgery like that would be expensive. We had finally saved enough money to take a vacation to visit my cousin in Florida during the summer. The trip would be a celebration trip since both boys would be graduating college in May. I decided that Chris should have some say in what we would do. Chris was home on spring break so we shared the news with him. When I asked, "What if the surgery costs so much money that we can't go visit Kate, would you still want Zelda to have the surgery?" Chris said, "Yes." Then I asked him, "What if Robert decides to go ahead with our vacation plans?" Chris said sadly, "Let's find out how much the operation will cost. If it's not more than $800 let's go ahead with it. But I want to go with you to see the surgeon when I come home in May."

Since I was very weak again and getting IV steroids, my mother offered to come to help again. Prior to my recent symptoms I wrote the menu of dinner meals for the week. Usually each weekend I decide what meals I will cook for dinner for the upcoming week. Then Howie does the food shopping. Because I teach and don't have any opportunity to make personal phone calls while at work, Howie often talks to my mother. I told him to tell her that we have food in the house to make meals. She could make any of the meals I planned, make her own meals, or buy out. While I was explaining that to Howie I was pointing to the dinner menu. I showed him that I had planned to make spaghetti on Friday because he likes to have the leftovers for lunch on Saturday. Howie stuck his lower lip and like a disappointed little boy pointed to Thursday's meal. It was sloppy Joes. He loves sloppy Joes. So he said, "What happened to that meal?" I responded defensively and with a tone of humor, "Well I had a little relapse!" Thankfully the Lord helped me make the sloppy Joes for him. I even made liver for him another night as a way of showing my appreciation for all he did for me. He loves liver but I can't imagine why. It's the most slimy, disgusting meat. It meant a lot to him when I made that.

Shortly after I finished the steroids I was supposed to grade the Praxis tests for Educational Testing Service (ETS). Those are the tests that college students preparing to become teachers must take and pass to get their teaching certifications. I had done it before with my good friend, Terry. It was good money for working during the weekend. I told Terry I didn't think I could go with her to grade the Praxis tests that weekend, since my neurologist said that any undue mental or physical stress could weaken me further. She responded that grading the tests wasn't really any stress at all. We simply sit and grade tests all day. The training ETS provides is good. In addition, they provide frequent breaks so that the teachers grading the tests get regular rests from the tedious concentration. I still didn't think I was up to it or that it was wise for me to do it. But I valued her opinion. She knew me and she knew the Praxis tests. I knew she would never advise me to do anything that wouldn't be good for me. That Friday, the day before the Praxis scoring, we didn't have school because it snowed quite a bit. I decided if I simply rested the entire day, I'd be able to do the Praxis scoring.

During the weekend my head was still spinning and I was still weak but I was able to do the scoring. But Sunday evening I was extremely tired. I was so listless that I was barely able to talk. When I'd tell people that I was tired they'd respond with a sympathetic nod and maybe with an added comment like, "Don't worry, Vicki. We're all tired. This is a busy time at school." It was frustrating not being able to explain my level of fatigue. I wanted people to understand my level of weakness so they wouldn't think that I was accepting all the help because I was simply tired. A dying plant drooping over might be a good picture of my fatigue. A toy running on a battery that is quickly running out of energy might help people understand that my reserve of energy had completely been depleted. Perhaps anyone who has had an operation has experienced the completely wiped out feeling you get right after surgery. I felt totally drained of life.

One day Howie and I went to pick up one of our cars. It simply needed an oil and lube. Howie looked at me and said, "I wish it was as easy to fix you. Maybe we could get you a new battery—perhaps a Die Hard." I told him, "That's one of the nicest things anyone has ever said to me." Howie had an idea how weak I was. He saw me struggle to climb our stairs. He'd watch me struggle to find the energy simply to stand up. That's why he appreciated my making dinner for him. He knew that it was an expression of love. His understanding helped me with my own acceptance.

My way of dealing with the disease was usually to go through the motions without thinking about it. By that I mean, there's a way to experience something unpleasant without reflecting on it. Going to the dentist is a good example. I hate going to the dentist. I even have a fear of dentists. So I don't go often. But when I have to go I don't think about it. I don't worry about what he might do. I force myself not to think about the awful sound of the drill. Writing this book, however, requires me to reflect on everything about the disease: my emotions, my symptoms, my experiences. This is truly a labor of love for people I'll never meet. There is a need for MS patients to find hope in the midst of uncertainty. I know that the Lord offers real hope. I know that many of you know the hope we find in the Bible. But we all need to be reminded of that hope.

I'm forcing myself to write this book as quickly as possible because I'm currently having a relapse. My arms and legs are weak. There is pain in my right leg—especially if I stay in one position for too long. My hands are also weak. So, I am writing it while I still can. I don't know if I'll get paresthesia again. If I did (which could happen tomorrow), that would prevent me from typing. I don't think I'm being unusually paranoid. I just think that this is life with MS. We have to be prepared for whatever may come our way. That's my form of acceptance for now.

Acceptance comes easier the more you know about God. He is a loving Father. He is a sovereign God who works all things for good. In the book of Romans we read, "And we know that all things work together for good to those who love God, to those who are the called according to His purpose." (Romans 8:28) In the book of Matthew we read about our loving Father. "'Ask, and it will be given to you; seek and you will find; knock, and it will be opened to you. For everyone who asks receives, and he who seeks finds, and to him who knocks it will be opened. Or what man is there among you who, if his son asks for bread, will give him a stone? Or if he asks for a fish, will give him a serpent? If you then, being evil, know how to give good gifts to your children, how much more will your Father who is in heaven give good things to those who ask Him!'" (Matthew 7:7-11)

If you truly believe that you are a child of the King, then you have access to His power and love. There is comfort in that. Resting in that knowledge might be difficult to do. It's only when we keep our focus on Him that we see how big He is. I learn from my students how I must seem to God. At the beginning of a school day one of my students walked hesitantly toward the classroom door but didn't come in. He waited at the door. As I walked toward him I could see him fighting back tears. He was a student who never cried. Before I asked him what was the matter he blurted out, "My yellow homework folder ripped so my mom gave me my sister's old folder." He showed me the folder and it was obviously a folder for a little girl. Everyone in the class had a yellow folder they used for homework. To my student this was a crisis that was impossible to fix. To me, it was simple to fix. I took the folder from his hand and laid it in the hallway so neither of us had to walk into the room holding the folder. I told him that I would take care of it. What he didn't know was that I keep extra yellow folders for occasions like that. I got a new yellow folder for him, put his name on it, and called him into the hallway. I presented the new folder to him and used the situation to teach him an important spiritual lesson. "To you this seemed like a big problem. But to me, it was just a little problem. In your life you will have very big problems. You need to remember that to God even your biggest problems are simple problems. He is an all powerful God. Always remember the folder." My prayer is that I will always remember that my MS (and all the problems that are caused by it) is a small problem for God to handle.

I've learned other similar lessons from my students. One day a parent volunteering in my classroom told me that one of my students was shivering. I went to her and asked her if she was cold. She said, "Yes." I told her to go to the nurse. The nurse keeps extra clothes in her office (in case students throw up on their clothes or they need a change of clothes for another reason).

The girl returned looking very preppie. She had selected a sweatshirt with our school's logo on it. It happened to go well with the skirt she was wearing. I took her into the hall to teach her a spiritual lesson. I pointed out that if she doesn't tell me her problems I can't solve them. She may not have told me about being cold because she might have thought that there was no solution to the problem. I told her that when she grows up she will have bigger problems. The Bible tells us we will all have trials in life. Sometimes our problems seem so big we think there's no way they can be solved. But God is bigger than any problem. God can always find a way. His power is so great. We can't allow our limited understanding of His power to prevent us from asking Him for help. I encouraged her to always remember to turn to Him and ask for His help.

CHAPTER 8

LIFE HAPPENS

During the school year when I was first diagnosed with MS I had two relapses. The first relapse was during the months of November and December. The second relapse, which started in March, lasted at least two months also. The reason I'm not quite sure of its duration is because that spring our older son, Chris, struggled with his own health issues.

At that time, Chris was away at college just weeks away from graduation. Earning a college degree is quite an accomplishment for anyone. You could say that for Chris it would have been miraculous. In his junior year of high school he began his journey with mental illness. Just weeks before Christmas that year he began unraveling. His mind started racing until eventually he was out of touch with reality. Several months later and after a stay in the psychiatric unit of a hospital, he was diagnosed with schizoaffective disorder (a hybrid of schizophrenia and psychosis). After his release from the hospital he entered a partial care facility which was followed by home-bound instruction. He finished his junior year of high school on time. But the following year he came very close to another psychotic episode. Once again, God was faithful in helping us all through it. Chris graduated on time from high school. Amazingly, he was accepted to two colleges. He enrolled in Penn State's business program and lived away at college.

During college his health only became more of a challenge. In addition to taking medication for his mental illness, he began medication for psoriatic arthritis. His rheumatologist also diagnosed Chris as having an underactive thyroid. If all that wasn't enough, he suffered from two severely herniated discs in his lower back. After treating his pain with epidural shots, Chris decided to have back surgery. During the summer he had a laminotomy (a partial disc removal). In spite of all his conditions, Chris still managed to audition and get accepted into Penn State's Marching Blue Band. Anyone who has experienced back pain from severely herniated discs can just wonder in amazement at how Chris was able to march in a band under such pain. Juggling the demands of college and the band in the context of severe back pain, arthritis, a thyroid condition, and mental illness was simply incredible. His tolerance to pain seemed at times to be superhuman. His primary physician commented once, "Chris, do you feel pain?" Obviously he does feel pain just like the rest of us, but his focus and resolve are extraordinary. He's able to ignore it. His will to accomplish things is astounding.

That's what made it so heart wrenching when he began to unravel again only weeks before his college graduation. His psychiatrist had to take him off some of his medication for his mental illness because his liver levels were elevated. His body was reacting to something and his psychotropic medication might have been the cause. But when faced with the pressures of passing literally one more test in order to graduate without sufficient medication, Zelda's tumor, and my MS, he started to lose his clarity of thought. He also had to get around campus with a fractured foot he got when he slipped on ice.

I was in the midst of my second relapse. I could tell from his voice on the phone that he wasn't doing well. But he was four hours away at college. Fortunately, he was in communication with his psychiatrist (who was also four hours away from him). It amazed me that Chris somehow managed to reach out to us and to his psychiatrist when he was barely able to think clearly. He refused to come home reasoning, "It's my last few weeks at college."

Finally on Easter he admitted himself into the psychiatric unit of the local hospital. My husband and I visited him and could tell that he was incoherent. I struggled with the apparent injustice of it. Chris had gotten so far against all odds. Would God, who had been so faithful thus far, allow him to miss graduation? Would Chris have to face the reality of his younger brother graduating from college before him? (Rob was due to graduate from college with a major in neuroscience and a minor in music.) Chris is academically "gifted" but you can't pass a college final if your mind isn't clear. He was so close to earning a degree in business with a minor in computer science. He had just one more test to pass in order to graduate—just one test.

He was released from the hospital into our care. Since Howie had earned a Master's degree in business, he was able to tutor Chris. Against the advice of Chris's psychiatrist, Chris insisted on going back to college to take his final exam. He had been barely stabilized in the hospital before being released. His condition was not at all under control. It wasn't until six months after his hospitalization that all his medication was finally adjusted. It's a long process to titrate medication down and to gradually increase new medication. Only one medication can be introduced at a time in order to determine its effectiveness. But, days after he was released from the hospital he had to face a final exam.

Around that time I was scheduled to attend a women's retreat with the ladies from our church. I had a choice. I could either stay at home and sit by the phone waiting for a desperate call from Chris, or I could go on the retreat and leave Chris in God's care. I decided to trust that the same God who had been faithful before would faithfully care for my son during this time of great challenge in the midst of mental torment. But I didn't know what the outcome would be. Would it be God's will to have Chris manage to pass the test and graduate, or would it be God's will to have Chris fail the test and not graduate before his brother? The bigger question I had to answer was, would my faith in a loving God waver if Chris didn't pass his test.

To search the deep parts of my heart, I turned to the Bible. I chose to read about someone in the Bible who was facing tremendous peril and who still trusted God without knowing the outcome. Many of the familiar stories in the Bible teach us great lessons. But the greatest lessons they hold are when we reflect on how those familiar characters didn't know the end of the story like we do. I turned to the story of when God's people were seemingly trapped at the Red Sea with the Egyptian army closing in. Never before had any human witnessed a sea opening up to allow millions of people to walk across on dry land. Moses' words encouraged my heart as I read what he told the children of Israel. He said, "Do not be afraid. Stand still, and see the salvation of the Lord, which He will accomplish for you today . . . The Lord will fight for you, and you shall hold your peace." (Exodus 14:13-14) I took comfort in that as a word from God to be at peace because God is in control. I could rest in that knowledge—no matter what the outcome.

Thankfully and miraculously Chris did pass the test and graduate. It was such a time of rejoicing as we witnessed both our sons graduate from college that spring.

Since Chris and I both have health conditions that significantly impact our lives from time to time, we share a bond unlike most other mothers and sons. We can totally empathize with each other. We both have our own specialists (both having our own neurologist). We both have to have regular blood tests (both of us need our liver levels checked). We both take a lot of medication. We both need to take good care of ourselves (eat right, get enough rest, etc.). Even some of our symptoms are similar at times. For example, my MS has begun affecting my cognitive abilities. Likewise, it's difficult for Chris to think at times (especially if he's tired). It's been healing for Chris to share this journey with me. On one of my first visits to the neurologist I had to leave work and go directly to the appointment. That day Chris was volunteering at the school where I teach so we went directly to the appointment. I told Christ that he didn't need to come into the office; he could wait in the lobby or the car. But he said, "No, Mom, you've been there for me for so many years. I want to be there for you." Chris once asked me, "Do you feel like a prisoner in your body because of your disease?" I responded, "I'm sure anyone with a disability feels trapped and helpless at one time or another. Their disease prevents them from doing what they want to do from time to time. Life seems unpredictable and people often feel helpless. But I don't feel helpless because my future is certain. Nothing is a surprise to God. God knows my future. Even if I can't do something—even if I have to stop teaching—I know that His plan for my life is perfect." I felt blessed to be in a situation where I could answer my son's completely honest question. He couldn't say, "Yea, that's easy for you to say." He knew that my words were spoken in the context of having an illness that isn't fun (to say the least!).

I debated whether or not to include the whole story about my son in this book about my MS. I decided to share those events because many people who struggle with MS do so in the context of other trails. A normal reaction to being struck with several trials at one time is to question God. I once attended an MS workshop where I met a married couple who had every reason to question God. They both had MS. After sharing the news that they both had MS, they said, "Yes, we were hit with a double whammy." Having MS is not our choice. We didn't cause our disease and it certainly wouldn't be our choice to live a life in the context of its symptoms. Our illness sometimes disrupts our short term plans and can even sabotage our long term goals. But it is our choice how we react to that fact. I told that couple about my son's illness and shared my perspective that, in a way, it's a blessing that we both have a disease. We can understand and empathize with each other. We know each other's struggles and can feel what it's like to face the challenges and disappointments that accompany a chronic illness. We share a bitter sweet dimension to our relationship.

CHAPTER 9

THE "MS GAME"

The next school year I had a relapse again in November. By that time I was familiar with the whole procedure. A nurse visited our home to insert a heplock into my hand for the Solu-Medrol treatments (IV steroids). Then Howie would administer each dose. The previous year my very first IV steroid treatments were administered four times each day: 6:00 AM, noon, 6:00 PM, and midnight ("6-12-6-12"). This year I wanted to go to work even with the heplock in my hand. My seven and eight year old students wouldn't understand why I was out for any length of time. I knew that the headmaster of our school would provide a substitute to be in with me so that I could teach without having to do all the physically demanding parts of the job. I could stay off my feet. So, I negotiated with my neurologist to reduce the amounts of doses from four doses to only three doses each day (for the three days of treatments). That eliminated a midday treatment which, in my words, 'wasn't very convenient.' My neurologist was starting to understand me better. He realized that I was happiest when I was with my students. Although he recommends to all his MS patients to stay as active as possible, he informed me that people having a relapse and being treated with IV steroids do not continue working. They are sometimes hospitalized. Reluctantly, however, he allowed me to go to work under the condition that I would be getting sufficient help (driving to work, having helpers at school, etc.).

One of the main reasons I felt compelled to go to work in spite of feeling completely drained of life was that many of my students that year were facing very serious life issues themselves. It was important to me to convey a message of hope to them. I wanted to tell them that I had MS and that I was at peace with the situation. God had given me an opportunity to teach a lesson that many of them needed.

What could a second grader be facing that's all that bad? Well, two of my students had a parent who had been treated for cancer a couple of years before. The prognosis for both of them was that the cancer would return and that the doctors wouldn't be able to cure them. They would die young (unless God healed them). Another boy's mother had been treated for breast cancer. So he, too, was aware that his mother might get cancer again and might not survive. A fourth student was related to a former student in our school who died of cancer when she was only in third grade. That fourth student also had an uncle who was being treated for cancer during the year she was in my class. So, four of my students were facing the possibility of the death of a close family member.

Other students in that class were facing equally significant trials. One of the boys had a potentially life-threatening allergy to dairy products. He couldn't have the same ice cream or the same pizza the other children could. He couldn't have most of the same treats all the other students had. His mother sent in treats that were safe for him and he'd select a treat from his special box of goodies. He also had asthma.

At the end of the year the students were in the sanctuary practicing for their spring concert and that boy looked like he was having trouble breathing. The pews had recently been treated with wood polish. The chemical was causing him to have an allergic reaction. Had he not been removed from the sanctuary immediately, he would have needed critical emergency medical care. His doctor said that he wouldn't be able to enter the sanctuary for the remainder of the school year (since the chemical fumes would still be in the air). This meant that the boy would miss the spring concert, the last two chapels, and the field day pep rally. I couldn't believe this was happening to the same boy who couldn't eat dairy products all the other children enjoyed.

By the way, I arranged to bring the chapels and pep rally to him. At our school, which is also a very large church, we have a separate room for nursing mothers. That small room has a closed circuit TV for the mothers to view the services on Sundays. I squeezed my whole class into that room during the chapels and pep rally.

The students could be part of a powerful illustration of God's perfect plan. At first it seemed like a terrible thing for that boy to be excluded from the sanctuary. But God used that situation to help him feel very special and loved by everyone. Since we were watching the chapels and pep rally from another location, the entire elementary student body gave a "shout out" to us. Instead of feeling sorry for himself, he felt highly valued and special. It was a powerful reminder of God's sovereignty for all those students living in uncertain situations. God can use even sad situations and make wonderful things happen.

Therefore, many of us in the classroom could ask the familiar question, "Why, God?" That's the question I wanted to answer. I hadn't told the students that I had MS yet, so I knew it was time to tell them. To prepare my lesson plan I pulled out the coloring book, *At Our House*, published by the National MS Society used to explain MS to children. As I flipped through the pages I realized that I didn't need to use the coloring book to develop my lesson. I was certainly an expert about the disease and didn't need to use any other resource to plan my lesson. God had prepared me to share about affliction and about His love.

The following is my lesson plan.

MS—A Lesson For Second Graders

Introduction: "I have some sad news to tell you and a lot of good news to share."

Explanation of the Disease:

- Attention Getter:

    Share some of my fun toys (brain bean bags, a toy that lets you push up a lever and a lolly pop brain pops up out of a man's head).

- Role Play the central nervous system. Explain that my immune system is "a little confused"—hurting good cells in my brain.
- Explanation:

    1. my symptoms (feel like a "wet noodle/kinda floppy", etc.)
    2. what could happen
    3. causes (not contagious)
    4. how it's diagnosed (show MRI)

The Truth:

When you don't know why something is happening, hold onto what you *do* know. We do know:

- God is in control.
- God has a perfect plan for my life.
- God will provide all that I need.

    1. strength
    2. wisdom
    3. helpers (When children fall down at recess other children come over to help. It's like a love attack. That's what it's like with

believers. God uses other Christians to help. It's like a love attack.)

Mv reactions:

- thankful: When you learn about something sad, count your blessings. There are always blessing to count. I am thankful . . .

  1. for protection—Since I have too many lesions to count on my brain, God protected my brain so that I'm not more disabled.
  2. for medicine—I'm thankful that there's medicine to slow down the progression of my disease.
  3. for my husband—"What do you think I say when he gives me my shot every other day?" I say, 'Thank you' because I'm thankful he loves me enough to help me."
  4. for the ability to see, to walk, to talk, etc.

- sad (when I can't be at school with my students)

The Bible:

- Discuss: Why did God allow it? Refer to lessons learned about why God allowed the plagues (to reveal His power). How can God show His power through Mrs. Chandler's MS?
- Romans 15:13

  "Now may the God of hope fill you with all joy and peace in believing, that you may abound in hope by the power of the Holy Spirit."

- We know God loves us because the Bible tells us so, not because of how things feel or seem. Song to reinforce that (sung slowly): Jesus Loves Me

Questions and Answers:

Video:

National MS Society's video: *Timmy's Journey to Understanding MS*

Reinforcement Activity:

National MS Society's coloring book, *At Our House*

Writer Response: (the following day—using only a word bank and not the information organizer poster)

Finish the following three statements:

1. MS is . . . .
2. God allowed Mrs. Chandler to have MS because . . .
3. I learned that whenever things are very sad or are very hard . . .

The initial lesson lasted about an hour. The students were appropriately concerned. They enjoyed the role playing portion of the lesson and got immediately quiet as I began to share the facts of the disease, especially my symptoms. Their solemn looks told me that they not only understood but were sympathetic. Their questions were insightful. But I wasn't sure they would remember the lesson or even be able to apply the truths I presented. My prayer was that God would write it on their hearts and minds. We all will face trials during our lives, but many of my students were facing serious trials as eight year old children. I needed to know if they understood that my situation could relate to theirs. So, that's why I had them complete three statements the following day. As I poured over their responses I could tell that they indeed comprehended it all. Thankfully they learned a lesson that was given to me by a loving Father to be shared with my students who were facing difficult life situations.

Shortly after that lesson the students had to have indoor recess (since it was raining outside). The recess aide told me after recess that my class was playing the "MS Game." She explained that they were acting out the central nervous system. Children take their cue from adults. I was so grateful that God used me to be an example of faith in action. Shots are no fun. It stinks to have MS. But God loves us and He is faithful . . . and it's fun to play the "MS Game."

CHAPTER 10

RICKETY VICKI

As we all know, life goes on for MS patients. Difficulties and trials come and go in the context of MS. That means we need to learn to manage the physical and emotional demands of life in spite of the constraints our disease creates. We need to get creative in how we use our resources (our time, other people's help, our energy, our money). My neurologist told me that physical and emotional stress will weaken me further. The weakening of my frame can lead to emotional stress (when it prevents me from doing what I want to do). So it's potentially a vicious cycle.

MS has a way of making it painfully obvious that we're not in control. But, actually, we all live with the myth of certainty. Only one thing is certain. God knows what will happen in our lives. MS patients, like everyone else, have to face difficulties with family members, challenges of work situations, major disappointments, moving, betrayals, significant life events (death of a loved one, divorce, etc.), and even additional sickness.

Taking interferon treatments requires periodic blood tests to check liver levels. When my alkaline phosphate levels kept elevating my neurologist was concerned. First he had me reduce the dosage of my interferon from high dose to low dose. Still the levels kept rising slightly. A gastrointestinal specialist concluded that my liver was fine. A blood test revealed that the elevated alkaline phosphate level was related to a bony structure. So, onto my primary physician I went. An x-ray and a bone density scan revealed that I had osteopenia. That didn't explain the elevated liver level or the constant pain I was experiencing deep in my forearms, thighs, or hips. Walking up just one step caused me pain. No matter what position I was in the pain was there. I attributed it to my MS until I realized that it might be caused by another condition.

Since I had just turned 50 years old I was also going through perimenapause. I was put on medication for the osteopenia. Incidentally the dreaded hot flashes seemed to pale in comparison to MS aches and my other constant pain. I guess that was kind of an advantage. But there was a bit of good news coming.

The next step was to see an endocrinologist. More tests were prescribed. The favorite tests doctors like to prescribe are blood tests. This specialist also prescribed a bone scan and more blood tests. I hate to be stuck by anything sharp. My veins are so small people often cannot easily locate them or need to use a baby needles. I feel like a human pin cushion!

Finally I received a diagnosis. I had osteomalacia (also known as Rickets when diagnosed in children). It results from a vitamin D deficiency. I told the doctor that my diet includes regular amounts of products that contain vitamin D. She informed me that a lack of sunshine could also cause the deficiency. Certainly that could be the case with me. Since the heat of the sun increases the pain of my aches, I avoid it.

Osteomalacia causes bone pain and fatigue. So why was it good news that I had been diagnosed with it? It can't be cured but it can be treated with high doses of Vitamin D. The good news is that the treatments which result in normal alkaline phosphate levels might also result in reduced pain and less fatigue. Prior to this new diagnosis I was resigned to the fact that my pain was part of life with MS. Now there was hope that much of the pain would subside.

When I came home I boasted to Chris, "Well now I also have three conditions, just like you." He inquired about the newest diagnosis. With appropriate concern and compassion he asked, "What is osteomalacia?" He wanted to know how I got it. I explained that I probably got the condition because of lack of sunshine. Without missing a beat he said, "You gotta get out more!"

A final note: After months of high dose vitamin D treatments, I still have the constant pain. I'm still "Rickety Vicki." Apparently it can take as long as two years to see some improvement, if any. By the way, I do realize that with osteomalacia and osteopenia my bones are not in good shape. I guess I'm more prone to fractures. Do you think it's a good idea to have MS—a disease which could impair my balance—along with those other two conditions? No! But I'm not the one who decided that I have all three conditions (and God does just fine making His own decisions without my help). So, OK, OK, I got it . . . "Take it easy." But that's a bit out of my comfort zone.

CHAPTER 11

WHEN A RELAPSE ISN'T THE WORST PART

Journaling has helped me identify patterns. For example, I realized that when I'm tapering off IV steroids and taking my Provigil (medication to give me energy) I get migraines. Once I'm off the oral taper I can resume the Provigil free of headaches.

When I got a relapse two years in a row in November I asked my neurologist if I caused them. That's an incredibly busy time of year for me. In addition to preparing for Thanksgiving dinner and shopping for Christmas gifts, I have to prepare for parent-teacher conferences and do report cards (in addition to teaching and grading papers). I also do things like take a weekend workshop or work an additional job over one weekend around that time (grading the Praxis tests). So I asked my neurologist if I can cause a relapse. He told me that I couldn't. However, by the time I got a relapse the third year in a row my neurologist knew me better.

One Wednesday in the middle of November I experienced some vision problems. It was at the end of the day. The students had just been dismissed. I was straightening up my classroom and preparing to go to our weekly faculty meeting. I noticed that everything looked like I was seeing it under glittery water. I had been feeling more tired but chalked it up to the fact that I had recently attended a weekend workshop. I told myself that anyone would be tired if they worked 12 days in a row. But deep down inside I was concerned that I might be heading into another relapse. I realized that my hazy vision could be signaling a relapse. I wondered if my vision was about to go at that moment. MS patients know that any symptom that accompanies a relapse can either be temporary (and leave when the relapse is over) or permanent. I realized that if my vision were to go completely I might not see again.

Thankfully, the episode lasted only about 30 mins. I had a regular appointment scheduled with my neurologist a week from then, so I didn't call him. I thought I'd mention it to him at the appointment and ask him to prescribe oral steroids since the vision problem probably meant there was inflammation near my optic nerve.

A week later I was still tired—probably more tired than I was admitting to myself. But by that time everyone around me was noticing that I was not myself. It was harder for me to think. I simply added that to the list of symptoms I'd speak to my neurologist about. I still was in a bit of denial about having a relapse. I looked around and saw how tired all the other teachers were after having parent-teacher conferences and writing report cards. In spite of my weakness, I told my principal that I'd like to teach an after school computer workshop for parents and their children. My principal responded by saying, "No you may not. I'm about to tell you not to come back after the two day Thanksgiving break, and to stay home until after Christmas vacation." She added that other teachers were concerned about me. I promised to rest over the Thanksgiving vacation and was allowed to return. I was grateful for her concern for my health.

When I went to the appointment with my neurologist I came prepared with my most recent MRI films and my list of questions. Chris waited in the car this time. I wasn't prepared for what I was about to hear. Had I known what my neurologist would say I would have asked my husband to accompany me to the office (since he was more than willing to take off from work any time to go with me). I shared with my neurologist all my symptoms, the comments of my principal, and my new MRI films. Then I asked him if I should be put on oral steroids. He said, "I do think it's a good idea to start you on Solu-Medrol." I asked him why I should begin IV steroids rather than oral steroids. He responded that he felt that if we treated this relapse aggressively it might be minimized. Hearing his acknowledgment of my relapse shook me out of my denial. I wasn't happy to face the reality of having to get a heplock in my hand, to possibly have to miss school, or to face getting symptoms that might not go away. But that wasn't the worst part of the visit.

I knew that this relapse might be considered proof the other teachers needed to convince me that I cause my relapses. So I said, "Everyone is going to tell me that I brought this relapse on myself. I just need you to tell me again that I can't cause my relapses." He responded by saying, "That's what I told you before because that's what I tell all my MS patients. But you're not like all my other MS patients. You keep the hours that I keep and I'm exhausted and I don't have MS. We know that if someone doesn't get sufficient sleep and rest it can affect the immune system. We also know that if you do that over years it can lead to heart disease or even cancer. You do have a disease of the immune system. So, yes, I do believe that you at least contributed to this relapse or caused it." That statement shocked me. I didn't see that coming. That was a life-changing statement. That meant I needed to make big changes. I couldn't do everything I wanted to. It didn't mean that I needed to quit teaching. It just meant that I could no longer work on weekends during the school year. I knew it meant that I couldn't do things like write books over vacations (like I'm doing now). But I knew it would take me some time to change old habits. It really meant I had to change part of who I am. I tend to obsess. For the sake of my health, that had to stop. But that still wasn't the worst part of the appointment.

I told him at previous appointments that I believed the MS was causing cognitive difficulties. It was harder for me to process things and there were times I couldn't recall a word. He usually pointed out that my older age could be the cause. To that I'd remark, "OK, we're done here." But just before that visit with him I attended an MS workshop where I learned new information. A neurologist from Duke University told a large audience of MS patients and their guests that we used to think that MS *could* cause cognitive difficulties; but we now know that MS *will* cause cognitive difficulties for every MS patient. The speaker acknowledged the fact that everyone in the large room was nodding their heads. We all were experiencing that symptom to some extent. It was evident to me that I, too, might experience some sort of impairment. I might have trouble with attention, processing, word retrieval, or memory. I just didn't know how pervasive my problems would be, how severe, or how quickly I'd see them manifested.

Up until that appointment, part of me could stay in denial about any cognitive difficulties. At a weekend workshop I learned to design a web site. Over the Thanksgiving break I read a book. It was easy to hold onto the comforting words of my neurologist that I'm just getting older. So at the appointment I posed the question, "Do you think my MS is affecting my cognitive abilities?" His response was completely unexpected. He said, "Considering the amount of white matter you have on your brain, I'm not at all surprised that you're experiencing some cognitive difficulties." I recalled reading that medication for Alzheimer's patients is prescribed for MS patients. So I asked him if it would be good for me to start taking that medication. He said that he wanted me to begin taking Aricept. He'd give me a sample month supply to see how I'd respond to it. I assumed that the Aricept would slow down the progression of the cognitive impairments. But I was wrong. Since my MS is the cause of the cognitive difficulties, the Aricept might only help me think better. It would not slow the progression of MS that was affecting my thinking.

That was devastating news I hadn't been prepared to hear. MS has been called "the disease that keeps on taking." When people are asked,

"If you had to become handicapped, what would be the worst thing for you" most people respond by saying that losing their vision would be the worst. But most people never consider that losing their mind could be a possibility. That only usually happens to older people. But I was just told that I was quite literally losing my mind. Since I began my career teaching blind students I know that people can learn to live and work with blindness. I know that people who lose their mobility can work and even drive. But you can't work with diminished ability to think.

At the end of the appointment I had a lot to remember without Chris (since he was waiting in the car). I had to carry my MRI films, get the Aricept sample, make an appointment for a follow-up visit (checking to see if I'd need a new referral), get the prescription for regular blood work (and a copy of it since the standing order somehow can't be located when I go for the blood tests), and get what I'd need for the steroids (Solu-Medrol prescription, the Prednisone oral steroids prescription, the Pepcid prescription to prevent stomach discomfort, and directions for the oral taper).

When I was in the elevator leaving the medical building I remembered that the doctor hadn't given me the Aricept sample. As I walked back to his office, I realized the irony of it. I had to laugh as I told the nurses, "I came back because I remembered that Dr. Mazlin didn't give me the sample of the medicine I need to help me think. Does that mean I don't get it now? They got a good laugh about it too. Dr. Mazlin does work very hard. He came out of his office handing me the sample apologizing, "I'm sorry. I forgot to give this to you." I told him that perhaps he needed it more than me!

That night while telling my husband all the information from my appointment I had a good cry. It's important to grieve losses—even the loss of faculties. The next day I was going to work—relapse and all. It was especially hard to think of all the details. The students were practicing for their Christmas program so the schedule was changed. There were so many details to hold in my head. But while I was getting ready for work a thought popped into my head. I got the idea to type a quick note to the parents of my students to let them know about several important things. I titled the memo: Three Points of Passion. I'm passionate about Penn State (since my mother and Chris graduated from there), learning, and the Lord. I wanted to let the parents know about a "Penn State Day" that I was planning for the class (since Penn State's football team tied first place in the Big Ten division). I also wanted to let the parents know about our new slogan, "Let the quest continue!" I introduced that slogan so the students would view learning as something that doesn't end at the end of the school day or at the end of graduation. It continues throughout life. Finally, I wanted to let them know a bit of my lesson to the students about MS. I realized that there was no way for the parents to know about the hope I conveyed in that lesson unless I told them. After I finished typing that note, I was off to work. While driving in the car, I was amazed at how the Lord was helping me remember every detail of the upcoming day. My thoughts shifted to the letter I typed. I was even more amazed that the Lord gave me the idea for the Three Points of Passion in the midst of my cluttered thinking. I whispered, "Thank you, Lord." That's when He spoke to my heart saying, "Vicki, I'll think for you." God is so gracious to provide assurance when we need it most. I hadn't even gotten to the place in my grieving where I cried out for peace and assurance. But God knows our every need even before we ask it. Mercifully, He provided that assurance before I went into despair.

I was losing my mind but not my sense of humor. When I told the staff the news their expressions were appropriately solemn. So I told them, "Why do you all look so glum? It's not your fault. You didn't cause it by 'picking my brain.'" Nowadays I'd be happy for someone to 'give me a piece of their mind.'

CHAPTER 12

PLANS FOR THE FUTURE?

Is it possible to make plans for the future when you have MS? That's a question we all have to ask. We know that we face uncertainty about our health. But the truth is that everyone's future is uncertain. There is a myth of certainty. At any moment a person's life could change. In an instant a car accident might leave an individual paralyzed. In a matter of seconds someone could be burned in a house fire. Aside from unexpected health problems, anyone could face a sudden change in finances (e. g., being fired). It is only by God's grace that any of us go through a period of time without a crisis.

So what is certain? His love is certain. God is never changing. He holds the details of our lives in the palm of His hand. We are called to live our lives looking unto Him. "Therefore we also, since we are surrounded by so great a cloud of witnesses, let us lay aside every weight, and the sin which so easily ensnares us, and let us run with endurance the race that is set before us, looking unto Jesus . . ." (Hebrews 12:1-2a) If I focus more on my MS then I begin to think about all the things that might happen. But if I focus more on the Lord then I seek His guidance for my future.

It's wonderful to think about all the research that is going on. But my confidence can't be in men. It has to be in the Lord who can provide the peace and wisdom that I need now. I can't wait for a cure to live my life. I can't put my life on hold to discover the purpose God has for me. Even if my disease causes me to stop working, I can have an assurance that God can still use me. I can always pray for others while lying in bed. I can encourage others on the phone if I'm too weak to leave home. Someone once said that all God needs is your availability not your ability. So even when we are unable to do much, God still has a plan for us.

The times we need to rest provide opportunities to read God's Word. Suddenly in the business of life God provides a season of fellowship with Him. The mistake MS patients might make is to hope there will be no more relapses. If you can expect to have them, then you might be able to accept them when they come.

That leads to the big question: can you accept whatever God has planned for your life? This might require flexibility beyond what you're comfortable with. That's one of the hardest things for me to deal with. I like to plan ahead. I don't like last minute changes to my plans. So when my disease causes me to unexpectedly change my course, I have a choice to make. I can either feel sorry for myself or remind myself that there are no surprises to God. He has an alternative plan for me. He allowed me to have the disease, He allows the relapses to come, and He will provide all the details of the adjustments that have to be made. I just need to trust Him more.

It's good to make plans for the future. Dr. Mazlin advises all his MS patients to stay as active as possible. But if we keep hold of our plans, determined not to let the MS interrupt them, we risk missing the plans God has for us. We need to be willing to switch plans—to yield to Him. The best place to be is in the center of God's will. How do you know what that means for your life? Ask God. He is a generous Father who promises to give us wisdom if we simply ask.

Your future will be brighter if you are prepared and informed. Pray for the best and plan for the worst. Be prepared by examining your financial situation (e. g., exploring other possible ways to earn money), insurance coverage, housing needs (e. g., considering what changes might need to be made to your home). Stay informed by reading all that the National MS Society sends you.

The question remains whether or not MS patients can make plans. Shortly after I was diagnosed with MS we wanted to make plans to visit my cousin in Florida. We made the plans. We bought the plane tickets. If the time comes for our vacation in Florida and I'm unable to go, then I'll deal with that at the time. We can always pray for wisdom to know what plans to make. We don't know what our future holds, but He does.

I challenge you to face your future with a new perspective. A new perspective involves meeting some new goals. Those goals are not achieved once and for all; they must be achieved daily (sometimes even minute by minute).

The Goals:

- Live with humor and faith.
- Focus on Him more than on the disease.
- Yield to His timing and plans.
- Cling to God's Word.

CHAPTER 13

HAVING A PURPOSE

Everyone wants to know that there's a purpose to their life. When MS causes you to stop working for a period of time or perhaps completely, you wonder what the point of your life is. MS can trigger an identity crisis. I've taught for about 25 years and I realize that I might have to reevaluate my role in life. I might have to redefine who I am. I am considering other more realistic options—things that I could do that wouldn't require so much energy if my MS prevents me from teaching. However, my heart always has been and still is in teaching.

When we face an identity crisis we ask, "Where do I fit in? Will I ever make a difference? What's the meaning of my life? What do I have to contribute? Am I needed?" MS can leave an individual without a clear calling or mission.

Some of the common mistakes individuals make in their search for purpose include:

- Aiming too high/having unrealistic aspirations—MS patients struggle to identify realistic aspirations for life. The unpredictability of the disease causes us to rethink our aspirations frequently (depending on the number and severity of our relapses). That can lead to frustration and discouragement.
- Deciding on a particular purpose for the wrong reasons (e. g., fame, fortune)
- Coveting another person's purpose or calling—saying. "I wish I could do that job."
- Ignoring your obvious calling
- Jumping from one purpose to another
- Waiting for a time later in life to consider a purpose—saying, "I'll deal with it when the time comes."

Perhaps the greatest mistake that people make is that they equate a successful job with purpose. It certainly is an accomplishment to be successful in your job, however you can have a calling in life without even being employed.

* * *

A job is a means to live.
A purpose is the meaning of one's life.

So, what can produce a genuine feeling of purpose? A calling can be either temporal (as in the case with most occupations) or of eternal value. Those that have eternal value serve a supportive function, for the benefit of others. Usually those roles are not as visible or as glamorous as many occupations. But those who understand the importance and value of a supportive function find far greater satisfaction than any job can provide. It is when we focus on serving others that we gain real fulfillment. Examples of supportive functions in life include:

- Raising godly children

    "Train up a child in the way he should go, and when he is old he will not depart from it." Proverbs 22:6

- Praying for others/being a faithful prayer warrior

    "And the Lord said to Moses, 'I have seen this people, and indeed it is a stiff-necked people. Now therefore, let Me alone, that My wrath may burn hot against them and I may consume them. And I will make of you a great nation.' Then Moses pleaded with the Lord his God, and said, 'Lord, why does Your wrath burn hot against Your people whom You have brought out of the land of Egypt with great power and with a mighty hand? Why should the Egyptians speak, and say, He brought them out to harm them, to kill them in the mountains, and to consume them from the face of the earth? Turn from Your fierce wrath, and relent from this harm to Your people. Remember Abraham, Isaac, and Israel, Your servants, to whom You swore by Your own self, and said to them, I will multiply your descendants as the stars of heaven; and all this land that I have spoken of I give to your descendants, and they shall inherit it forever.' So the Lord relented from the harm which He said He would do to His people." (Exodus 32:9-14)

(Imagine that! Moses interceded for a multitude of God's people and God changed His mind. Your prayers for others can make a difference.)

"For this reason we also, since the day we heard it, do not cease to pray for you . . ." (Colossians 1:9a)

". . . pray for one another, that you may be healed. The effective, fervent prayer of a righteous man avails much. Elijah was a man with a nature like ours, and he prayed earnestly that it would not rain; and it did not rain on the land for three years and six months. And he prayed again, and the heaven gave rain, and the earth produced its fruit." (James 5:16-18)

- Being a peacemaker

  "Blessed are the peacemakers, for they shall be called sons of God." (Matthew 5:9)

- Encouraging others

  "And I looked, and arose and said to the nobles, to the leaders, and to the rest of the people, 'Do not be afraid of them. Remember the Lord, great and awesome, and fight for your brethren, your sons, your daughters, your wives, and your houses . . . Therefore, wherever you hear the sound of the trumpet, rally to us there. Our God will fight for us.'" (Nehemiah 4:14, 20)

- Comforting others and showing compassion

  "Blessed be the God and Father of our Lord Jesus Christ, the Father of mercies and God of all comfort, who comforts us in all our tribulation, that we may be able to comfort those who are in any trouble, with the comfort with which we ourselves are comforted by God." (II Corinthians 1:3-4)

- Doing good works (visiting the sick, helping the poor, etc.)

  "For we are His workmanship, created in Christ Jesus for good works, which God prepared beforehand that we should walk in them." (Ephesians 2:10)

"This is a faithful saying, and these things I want you to affirm constantly, that those who have believed in God should be careful to maintain good works. These things are good and profitable to men." (Titus 3:8)

"But someone will say, 'You have faith, and I have works.' Show me your faith without your works, and I will show you my faith by my works. For as the body without the spirit is dead, so faith without works is dead also." (James 2:18, 26)

"My little children, let us not love in word or in tongue, but in deed and in truth." (I John 3:18)

- Evangelizing

  "And He said to them, 'Go into all the world and preach the gospel to every creature.'" (Mark 16:15)

  "To me, who am less than the least of all the saints, this grace was given, that I should preach among the Gentiles the unsearchable riches of Christ." (Ephesians 3:8)

- Listening and being a counselor

  "Have I not written to you excellent things of counsels and knowledge, that I may make you know the certainty of the words of truth, that you may answer words of truth to those who I send to you?" (Proverbs 22:20-21)

  "Counsel in the heart of man is like deep water, but a man of understanding will draw it out." (Proverbs 20:5)

  "He who has knowledge spares his words, and a man of understanding is of a calm spirit." (Proverbs 17:27)

- Bringing joy into the lives of others (sharing a smile, music, or art)

  "And so it was, whenever the spirit from God was upon Saul, that David would take a harp and play it with his hand. Then Saul would become refreshed and well, and the distressing spirit would depart from him." (I Samuel 16:23)

"For we have great joy and consolation in your love, because the hearts of the saints have been refreshed by you, brother." (Philemon 7)

- Loving the unlovely, lonely, or those rejected or ignored by others (the elderly, the handicapped, the homeless, the child without parents, the student who is unmercifully teased by others)

    "Then the righteous will answer Him, saying, 'Lord, when did we see You hungry and feed You, or thirsty and give You drink? When did we see You a stranger and take You in, or naked and clothe You? Or when did we see You sick, or in prison, and come to You?' And the King will answer and say to them, 'Assuredly, I say to you, inasmuch as you did it to one of the least of these My brethren, you did it to Me.'" (Matthew 25:37-40)

Notice that each supportive function has a biblical basis. Each of us has a God-given role in life and a calling. Simply pray and ask God to reveal to you what part you can play that will have eternal value. It is His good pleasure to guide you toward His purpose for you. You can make a difference in the lives of others—even with MS. Perhaps you are already fulfilling one or more of these roles and didn't appreciate the eternal value of it.

Regardless of the fact that you have a disease that weakens you, you can have a purpose. God's Word is full of assurances that He has a plan for His children. Read and meditate on the following verses until you believe that he has a calling for you.

- Our purpose is a holy calling.

    "Therefore do not be ashamed of the testimony of our Lord, nor of me His prisoner, but share with me in the sufferings for the gospel according to the power of God, who has saved us and called us with a holy calling, not according to our works, but according to His own purpose and grace which was given to us in Christ Jesus before time began." (II Timothy 1:6-9)

- One heavenly purpose is to equip the saints.

    "And He Himself gave some to be apostles, some prophets, some evangelists, and some pastors and teachers, for the equipping of the saints for the work of ministry, for the edifying of the body of Christ." (Ephesians 4:11-12)

- Weaker members have an important purpose.

  "But one and the same Spirit works all these things, distributing to each one individually as He wills. For as the body is one and has many members, but all the members of that one body, being many, are one body, so also is Christ. For by one Spirit we were all baptized into one body—whether Jews or Greeks, whether slaves or free—and have all been made to drink into one Spirit. For in fact the body is not one member but many. If the foot should say, 'Because I am not a hand, I am not of the body,' is it therefore not of the body? And if the ear should say, 'Because I am not an eye, I am not of the body,' is it therefore not of the body? If the whole body were an eye, where would be the hearing? If the whole were hearing, where would be the smelling? But now God has set the members, each one of them, in the body just as he pleased. And if they were all one member, where would the body be? But now indeed there are many members, yet one body. And the eye cannot say to the hand, 'I have no need of you'; nor again the head to the feet, 'I have no need of you.' No, much rather, those members of the body which seem to be weaker are necessary. And those members of the body which we think to be less honorable, on these we bestow greater honor; and our unpresentable parts have greater modesty." (I Corinthians 12:11-23)

- We are given a purpose before birth.

  "Before I formed you in the womb I knew you, and before you were born I consecrated you; I have appointed you a prophet to the nations. (Jeremiah 1:5)

- Another heavenly purpose is to love others and to be His disciples.

  "'A new commandment I give to you, that you love one another, even as I have loved you, that you also love one another. By this all men will know that you are My disciples, if you have love for one another.'" (John 13:34-35)

- God's purpose is for you to testify of the gospel.

"... in order that I may finish my course, and the ministry which I received from the Lord Jesus, to testify solemnly of the gospel of the grace of God." (Acts 20:24)

- God's purpose is to demonstrate God's power in you for the benefit of others.

  "For this purpose I raised you up, to demonstrate My power in you, and that My name might be proclaimed throughout the whole earth." (Romans 9:17)

- God's purpose is to put you into service.

  "I thank Christ Jesus our Lord, who has strengthened me, because He considered me faithful, putting me into service;" (I Timothy 1:12)

- God chooses you for a purpose.

  "Just as He chose us in Him before the foundation of the world that we should be holy and blameless before Him. In love He predestined us to adoption as sons through Jesus Christ to Himself, according to the kind intention of His will," (Ephesians 1:4-5)

- God predestined you and called you according to His purpose.

  "And we know that all things work together for good to those who are the called according to His purpose. For whom He foreknew, He also predestined to be conformed to the image of His Son, that He might be the firstborn among many brethren. Moreover whom He predestined, these He also called; whom He called, these He also justified; and whom He justified, these He also glorified." (Romans 8:28-30)

- God works His purpose through us.

  "Lord, You will establish peace for us, for You have also done all our work in us." (Isaiah 26:12)

There is a familiar expression regarding job seeking that says, "It's not what you know, but who you know." Sometimes it's true that a person will have a better chance at getting a job if he knows someone associated with the company who has some authority or influence. Credentials sometimes don't matter as much as recommendations. There is even greater validity to that statement when you consider God's role in providing a job or a purpose for your life. It's not what you know, but Who you know.

"A man's heart plans his way, but the Lord directs his steps."
(Proverbs 16:9)

CHAPTER 14

VERSES OF HOPE

Verses Regarding Physical Strength:

". . . 'My grace is sufficient for you, for My strength is made perfect in weakness.' Therefore most gladly I will rather boast in my infirmities, that the power of Christ may rest upon me. Therefore I take pleasure in infirmities . . . for Christ's sake. For when I am weak, then I am strong." (II Cointhians 12:9-10) "He gives power to the weak and to those who have no might He increases strength." "But those who wait on the Lord shall renew their strength; they shall mount up with wings like eagles. They shall run and not be weary. They shall walk and not faint." "Fear not, for I am with you. Be not dismayed, for I am your God. I will strengthen you. Yes, I will help you. I will uphold you with My righteous right hand." "For I, the Lord your God, will hold your right hand saying to you, Fear not, I will help you.'" (Isaiah 40:29-30) (Isaiah 41:10, 13)

"I can do all things through Christ who strengthens me." (Philippians 4:13)

"Finally, my brethren, be strong in the Lord and in the power of His might." (Ephesians 6:10)

". . . 'So I will save you, and you shall be a blessing. Do not fear. Let your hands be strong.'" (Zechariah 8:13b)

"The Lord will give strength to His people; the Lord will bless His people with peace." (Psalm 29:11)

"I will go in the strength of the Lord God . . ." (Psalm 71:16a)

"Seek the Lord and His strength; seek His face evermore." (Psalm 105:4)

"The Lord will strengthen him on his bed of illness; You will sustain him on his sickbed." (Psalm 41:3)

"For thus says the Lord God, the Holy One of Israel: 'In returning and rest you shall be saved; in quietness and confidence shall be your strength.' Therefore the Lord will wait, that He may be gracious to you; and therefore He will be exalted, that He may have mercy on you. For the Lord is a God of justice; blessed are all those who wait for Him." (Isaiah 30:15, 18)

"Yet I will rejoice in the Lord, I will joy in the God of my salvation. The Lord God is my strength; He will make my feet like deer's feet, and He will make me walk on my high hills." (Habakkuk 3:18-19)

"But may the God of all grace, who called us to His eternal glory by Christ Jesus, after you have suffered a while, perfect, establish, strengthen, and settle you." (I Peter 5:10)

"For this reason I bow my knees to the Father of our Lord Jesus Christ, from whom the whole family in heaven and earth is named, that He would grant you, according to the riches of His glory, to be strengthened with might through His Spirit in the inner man," (Ephesians 3:14-16)

"For this reason we also, since the day we heard it, do not cease to pray for you, and to ask that you may be filled with the knowledge of His will in all wisdom and spiritual understanding; that you may have a walk worthy of the Lord, fully pleasing Him, being fruitful in every good work and increasing in the knowledge of God; strengthened with all might, according to His glorious power, for all patience and longsuffering with joy;" (Colossians 1:9-11)

"For when we were still without strength, in due time Christ died for the ungodly." (Romans 5:6)

"Strengthen the weak hands, and make firm the feeble knees. Say to those who are fearful-hearted, 'Be strong, do not fear! Behold, your God will come with vengeance, with the recompense of God; He will come and save you.'" (Isaiah 35:3-4)

"Therefore strengthen the hands which hang down, and the feeble knees, and make straight paths for your feet, so that what is lame may not be dislocated, but rather be healed." (Hebrews 12:12-13)

* * *

Verses Regarding Inner Strength:

"I will love You, O Lord, my strength. The Lord is my rock and my fortress and my deliverer; my God, my strength, in whom I will trust; my shield and the horn of my salvation, my stronghold. I will call upon the Lord, who is worthy to be praised; so shall I be saved from my enemies." (Psalm 18:1-3)

"The Lord is my light and my salvation; whom shall I fear? The Lord is the strength of my life; of whom shall I be afraid?" (Psalm 27:1)

"Wait on the Lord; be of good courage, and He shall strengthen your heart; wait, I say, on the Lord!" (Psalm 27:14)

"For in YAH, the Lord is everlasting strength." (Isaiah 26:4)

"O Lord, my strength and my fortress, my refuge in the day of affliction . . ." (Jeremiah 16:19)

"Be of good courage, and He shall strengthen your heart, all you who hope in the Lord." (Psalm 31:24)

"O God, You are more awesome than Your holy places. The God of Israel is He who gives strength and power to His people." (Psalm 68:35)

"Blessed is the man whose strength is in You, whose heart is set on pilgrimage." (Psalm 84:5)

"Finally, my brethren, be strong in the Lord and in the power of His might." (Ephesians6:10)

Verses Regarding Affliction:

"For I consider that the sufferings of this present time are not worthy to be compared with the glory which shall be revealed in us." (Romans 8:18)

"In their affliction they will diligently seek Me." (Hosea 5:15)

"It is good for me that I have been afflicted, that I may learn Your statutes." (Psalm 119:71)

Good self talk for those with affliction:

"Why are you cast down, O my soul? And why are you disquieted within me? Hope in God, for I shall yet praise Him for the help of His countenance." (Psalm 42:5, Psalm 42:11, and Psalm 43:5)

"Unless Your law had been my delight, I would then have perished in myaffliction." (Psalm 119:92)

"And not only that, but we also glory in tribulations, knowing that tribulation produces perseverance; and perseverance, character, and character, hope. Now hope does not disappoint, because the love of God has been poured out in our hearts by the Holy Spirit who was given to us. For when we were still without strength, in due time Christ died for the ungodly. For scarcely for a righteous man will one die; yet perhaps for a good man someone would even dare to die. But God demonstrates His own love toward us, in that while we were still sinners, Christ died for us." (Romans 5:3-8)

"For those who live according to the flesh set their minds on the things of the flesh, but those who live according to the Spirit, the things of the Spirit. For to be carnally minded is death, but to be spiritually minded is life and peace." (Romans 8:5-6)

"Blessed be the God and Father of our Lord Jesus Christ, the Father of mercies and God of all comfort, who comforts us in all our tribulation, that we may be able to comfort those who are in any trouble, with the comfort with which we ourselves are comforted by God. For as the sufferings of Christ abound in us, so our consolation also abounds through Christ. Now if we are afflicted, it is for your consolation and salvation, which is effective for enduring the same sufferings which we also suffer. Or if we are comforted, it is for your consolation and salvation. And our hope for you is steadfast, because we know that as you are partakers of the sufferings, so also you will partake of the consolation." (II Corinthians 1:3-7)

Verses of Hope:

"I will bless the Lord who has given me counsel; my heart also instructs me in the night seasons. I have set the Lord always before me; because He is at my right hand I shall not be moved. Therefore my heart is glad, and my glory rejoices; my flesh also will rest in hope." (Psalm 16:7-9)

"You are my hope in the day of doom." (Jeremiah 17:17)

"'Call to Me, and I will answer you, and show you great and mighty things, which you do not know.'" (Jeremiah 33:3)

"Cast your burden on the Lord, and He shall sustain you; He shall never permit the righteous to be moved. (Psalm 55:22)

"And He said, 'My presence will go with you, and I will give you rest.'" "Then He said, 'I will make all My goodness pass before you, and I will proclaim the name of the Lord before you. I will be gracious to whom I will be gracious, and I will have compassion on whom I will have compassion.'" (Exodus 33:14, 19)

". . . so I will save you, and you shall be a blessing. Do not fear, let your hands be strong." (Zechariah 8:13b)

"Therefore I will look to the Lord; I will wait for the God of my salvation; My God will hear me. Do not rejoice over me, my enemy; when I fall, I will arise; when I sit in darkness, the Lord will be a light to me." (Micah 7:7-8)

"For I have satiated the weary soul, and have replenished every sorrowful soul." (Jeremiah 31:25)

"For consider Him, who endured such hostility from sinners against Himself, lest you become weary and discouraged in your souls." (Hebrews 12:3)

"I waited patiently for the Lord; and He inclined to me, and heard my cry. He also brought me up out of a horrible pit, out of the miry clay, and set my feet upon a rock, and established my steps. He has

put a new song in my mouth—Praise to our God; many will see it and
fear, and will trust in the Lord." (Psalm 40:1-3)

Verse For While You Are Shut-In Or Homebound:

- "I will behave wisely in a perfect way. Oh, when will You come to
  me? I will walk within my house with a perfect heart." (Psalm 101:2)
- "There is no fear in love; but perfect love casts out fear, because
  fear involves torment. But he who fears has not been made perfect
  in love. We love Him because He first loved us." (I John 4:18-19)

CHAPTER 15

GENERAL INFORMATION ABOUT MS

My Explanation of the Disease:

Throughout this book I've referred to the National MS Society. They truly are an excellent source of information about MS. Their booklets and flyers provide accurate information in easy to understand words. I strongly encourage those of you with MS to register with the society. Not only will you gain information about your illness, but you will support an organization that is actively working to find a cure for MS.

Rather than begin by quoting an explanation of MS from the National Society's booklets, I prefer to offer my own explanation. It's good practice to explain your disease. Many family members and friends will not completely understand MS and will want to further their knowledge. You are the expert about your disease, but it may not be easy for you to explain it. Here's the way I explain it.

Doctors and scientists believe that MS is an autoimmune disease. The immune cells in my brain are confused. Instead of fighting viruses, my immune cells attack perfectly good cells in my central nervous system. My immune system is overactive. Doctors believe that a virus might have caused my immune system to become overactive. Since I had an uncle who had MS, I was predisposed to get the disease.

When my immune system attacks my brain it damages the insulation or the mylen around the nerve cells in my brain. Each area that is damaged results in a lesion that can be seen on an MRI of the brain as a white spot. When lesions occur, all kinds of problems can result—depending on where the lesions occur. Since the brain controls all bodily functions, MS can impair things such as vision, speech, mobility, emotions, bladder control, cognitive ability (such as memory).

When the lesions are occurring, an MS patient might experience several symptoms, mild symptoms, or no symptoms at all. The attack is referred to a relapse, a flare, or an exacerbation. The relapse can last anywhere from several days to approximately six months. When the relapse is over, some of the symptoms might still remain or all of the symptoms could go away. **The course of the disease differs from patient to patient.**

There are some symptoms that many MS patients have in common. Extreme or acute fatigue is often associated with MS. The patient usually feels significantly exhausted or weak even during a time of remission when there are otherwise no other symptoms. Many MS patients experience depression at one time or another. In addition, many MS patients experience unusual sensations such as numbness in the extremities or parasthesia (a pins and needles feeling). Certain emotional responses are similar among most MS patients. The disease can cause feelings of frustration, fear, grief, (denial guilt, sadness), helplessness, anger, isolation, uncertainty, or confusion.

Most people have relapsing-remitting MS. That means they experience a relapse followed by a period of remission where they can appear perfectly fine. Many MS patients begin with relapsing-remitting MS and after about 10 years develop secondary-progressive MS. Secondary-progressive MS involves having fewer attacks with only partial recovery or no attacks but the symptoms and disabilities slowly become worse. There is another, more rare type of MS which is called primary-progressive MS. Those patients experience symptoms that do not remit and become worse. All of the types of MS may stabilize or become worse at any time. It is a disease that is not yet completely understood and therefore is difficult to predict.

Treatments for MS:

There is no cure for MS. However it can be treated. MS is treated in two ways. Medication, called disease-modifying drugs are prescribed to reduce the frequency and severity of the attacks. Those drugs which are interferons have proven to delay the onset of permanent disabilities (which are caused when nerve cells are not simply damaged, but destroyed). There are also many kinds of medications and treatments that effectively treat the symptoms of the disease. For example, physical therapy assists MS patients who have difficulty walking. Occupational therapy helps MS patients deal with fatigue or cognitive problems (teaching problem solving skills and life style changes). Even chemotherapy is being used with some MS patients.

Recently researchers found that the brain can repair itself, or remyelinate. But the remylenation occurs much slower than the demylenation (or damage to the insulation of the nerves). Many studies are being done to investigate possible cures and treatments for MS.

Suggestions:

- Apply for a handicapped parking permit. There will be times you'll need to conserve energy.
- Pray before you disclose you have the disease to people, especially to your employer.
- Be ready with an answer when people react to your illness. People who don't completely understand your disease may make comments or offer suggestions that are not helpful. You need to understand that they mean well and that's the way they show their concern. Be prepared to thank them for their sincere concern and prayers. When you are newly diagnosed you are still reacting to the news yourself. So, it's helpful to think of how you'll respond to information that is not accurate. If they share a story about someone else with MS who is "doing fine" and who is using some sort of alternative therapy, decide ahead of time how you'll respond to that. I usually say, "I'm glad she's doing fine. I don't know if that would work for me because MS differs from patient to patient. I'll speak to my neurologist about that. Thanks for your concern."
- Accept help. For someone, like me, relying on others is a very foreign experience. I choose to be independent. The fact is there will be times when I will need help. I'm learning to accept all the help that is freely offered to me. One fellow teacher pointed out that if I decline someone's offer to help me, I prevent them from receiving a blessing. People who love you want to do something to help you. So take them up on it.
- Make adjustments to your life style. MS will demand shifts in your life style. For example, I don't go up and down the steps in my house as often as I used to. I make lists of what I need to do downstairs and I wait until I have finished everything I need to do downstairs before going upstairs. When I pulled my back out I had to make similar adjustments. Instead of carrying my school bag over my shoulder, I now use a suitcase with wheels to transport my books. When my hands had parasthesia and were weak, I couldn't help my students tie their shoes, open things, or fix their zipper problems. I realized that there were some students in the class who were experts at opening things or tying shoes quickly. So I told them to help each other. Get creative or have someone help you brainstorm ways to solve your specific problems.

CHAPTER 16

PROTECTOR OF MY SOUL

"Unless Your law had been my delight, I would then have perished in my affliction." Psalm 119:92

Being a Christian with MS has to make a difference. If we trusted Jesus as our Savior, then we should trust Him as Lord in our lives. But we don't always know if we'd be able to have the trust we need in the face of tragedies. The good news is that when we go through the darkest valley God does all the work. He draws close to us. The Bible tells us God is near to those with a broken heart.

"The Lord is near to those who have a broken heart, and saves such as have a contrite spirit. Many are the afflictions of the righteous, but the Lord delivers him out of them all." Psalm 34:18-19

The Bible also tells us that Jesus' mission is to heal the brokenhearted.

"The Spirit of the Lord God is upon Me, because the Lord has anointed Me to preach good tidings to the poor. He has sent Me to heal the brokenhearted . . ." Isaiah 61:1

If you fear the worst, my dear partners in pain, be assured that the Lord will grant you the peace you need. I had the advantage of experiencing that first hand long before my diagnosis of MS.

When Chris was in his junior year of high school and became incoherent, suddenly the mind of a teenager with an IQ of 144 was gone. Suddenly my son was in torment, unstable, and non-communicative. For two months I was alone with him during the day witnessing a shattered life and bazaar behaviors. I couldn't sleep or leave him unsupervised. With a broken heart and no sleep, I had a supernatural calmness. Both peace and sorrow filled my heart. Chris's racing mind prevented me from having any conversation with him. I marveled at how the Lord could give me His peace while watching my son's agony. I wanted desperately to share the wonderful news that God **is** alive in me. The Holy Spirit comforted me and protected my soul when my heart was breaking for my son. I wanted everyone to know that we need not fear the worst. God is truly faithful. And He doesn't wait for us to pray the right prayer. He turns our tears into prayer. God gives us an example of that in Genesis. Hagar and her son were sent away in the Wilderness by Abraham. When the water supply dried up, Hagar resigned herself to the fact that her son would die of thirst.

> "And the water in the skin was used up, and she placed the boy under one of the shrubs. Then she went and sat down across from him at a distance of about a bowshot; for she said to herself, 'Let me not see the death of the boy.' So she sat opposite him, and lifted her voice and wept. And God heard the voice of the lad. Then the angel of God called to Hagar out of heaven and said to her, 'What ails you, Hagar? Fear not, for God had heard the voice of the lad where he is. Arise, lift up the lad and hold him with your hand, for I will make him a great nation.' And God opened her eyes, and she saw a well of water. Then she went and filled the skin with water, and gave the lad a drink. So God was with the lad; and he grew and dwelt in the wilderness, and became an archer." Genesis 21:14-20

A song came to my mind. I couldn't remember all the words. Only one particular part was the song of my heart. So I sang aloud:

> "Oh Holy Spirit, come,
> Show the world where life comes from
> May they always see You alive in me
> Oh Holy Spirit come."

Then I said aloud, mostly asking myself, "What's the rest of that song?" To my surprise Chris, proceeded to sing beautifully the entire song. What a gift!

> Oh, Protector of my soul,
> You will stand against the foe;
> In the dark You'll be a light for me,
> Oh, Protector of my soul.

Oh, gracious God above,
I could never earn Your love:
I'm amazed to see all You've given me,
Oh, gracious God above.

Chorus:
You, Who created the ends of the earth
Guided me unto Your throne;
Offered Your healing hand to me,
Mercif'lly made me Your own.

Oh, Holy Spirit, come,
Show the world where life comes from
May they always see you alive in me,
Oh, Holy Spirit, come.

Oh, Protector of my soul,
You will stand against the foe;
In the dark You'll be a light for me,
Oh, Protector of my soul.

The gift of trials is the blessed assurance that God is faithful. He comforts, protects, and carries us through our trials. He's the Good Shepherd caring for His sheep.

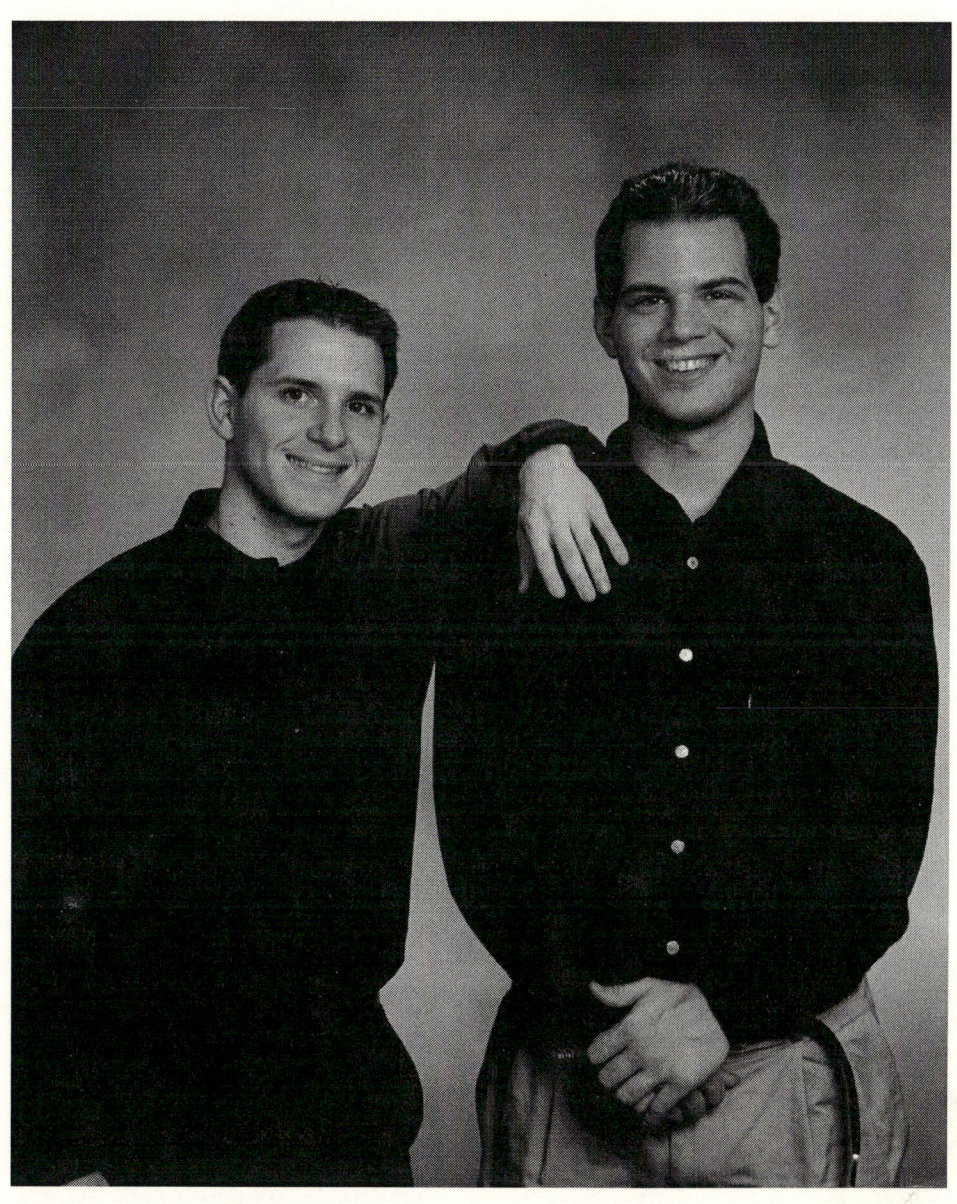

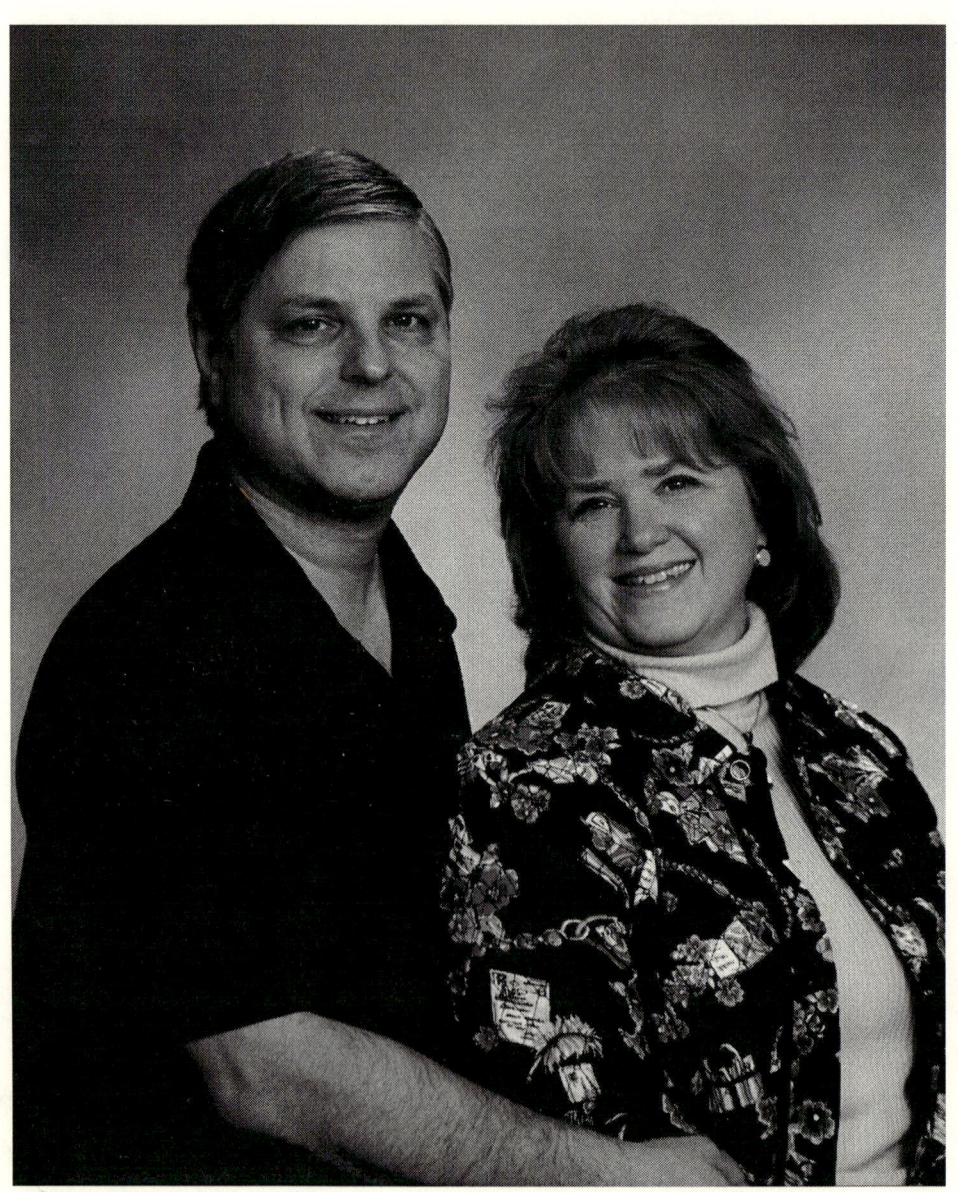